CN-55   CERTIFIED NURSE EXAMINATION SERIES

This is your
PASSBOOK for...

Certified Nursing Assistant

Test Preparation Study Guide
Questions & Answers

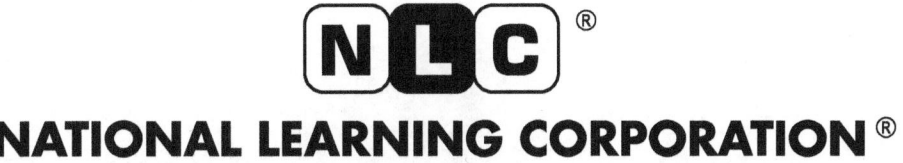

COPYRIGHT NOTICE

This book is SOLELY intended for, is sold ONLY to, and its use is RESTRICTED to individual, bona fide applicants or candidates who qualify by virtue of having seriously filed applications for appropriate license, certificate, professional and/or promotional advancement, higher school matriculation, scholarship, or other legitimate requirements of education and/or governmental authorities.

This book is NOT intended for use, class instruction, tutoring, training, duplication, copying, reprinting, excerption, or adaptation, etc., by:

1) Other publishers
2) Proprietors and/or Instructors of "Coaching" and/or Preparatory Courses
3) Personnel and/or Training Divisions of commercial, industrial, and governmental organizations
4) Schools, colleges, or universities and/or their departments and staffs, including teachers and other personnel
5) Testing Agencies or Bureaus
6) Study groups which seek by the purchase of a single volume to copy and/or duplicate and/or adapt this material for use by the group as a whole without having purchased individual volumes for each of the members of the group
7) Et al.

Such persons would be in violation of appropriate Federal and State statutes.

PROVISION OF LICENSING AGREEMENTS – Recognized educational, commercial, industrial, and governmental institutions and organizations, and others legitimately engaged in educational pursuits, including training, testing, and measurement activities, may address request for a licensing agreement to the copyright owners, who will determine whether, and under what conditions, including fees and charges, the materials in this book may be used them. In other words, a licensing facility exists for the legitimate use of the material in this book on other than an individual basis. However, it is asseverated and affirmed here that the material in this book CANNOT be used without the receipt of the express permission of such a licensing agreement from the Publishers. Inquiries re licensing should be addressed to the company, attention rights and permissions department.

All rights reserved, including the right of reproduction in whole or in part, in any form or by any means, electronic or mechanical, including photocopying, recording, or by any information storage and retrieval system, without permission in writing from the Publisher.

Copyright © 2024 by
National Learning Corporation

212 Michael Drive, Syosset, NY 11791
(516) 921-8888 • www.passbooks.com
E-mail: info@passbooks.com

PASSBOOK® SERIES

THE *PASSBOOK® SERIES* has been created to prepare applicants and candidates for the ultimate academic battlefield – the examination room.

At some time in our lives, each and every one of us may be required to take an examination – for validation, matriculation, admission, qualification, registration, certification, or licensure.

Based on the assumption that every applicant or candidate has met the basic formal educational standards, has taken the required number of courses, and read the necessary texts, the *PASSBOOK® SERIES* furnishes the one special preparation which may assure passing with confidence, instead of failing with insecurity. Examination questions – together with answers – are furnished as the basic vehicle for study so that the mysteries of the examination and its compounding difficulties may be eliminated or diminished by a sure method.

This book is meant to help you pass your examination provided that you qualify and are serious in your objective.

The entire field is reviewed through the huge store of content information which is succinctly presented through a provocative and challenging approach – the question-and-answer method.

A climate of success is established by furnishing the correct answers at the end of each test.

You soon learn to recognize types of questions, forms of questions, and patterns of questioning. You may even begin to anticipate expected outcomes.

You perceive that many questions are repeated or adapted so that you can gain acute insights, which may enable you to score many sure points.

You learn how to confront new questions, or types of questions, and to attack them confidently and work out the correct answers.

You note objectives and emphases, and recognize pitfalls and dangers, so that you may make positive educational adjustments.

Moreover, you are kept fully informed in relation to new concepts, methods, practices, and directions in the field.

You discover that you are actually taking the examination all the time: you are preparing for the examination by "taking" an examination, not by reading extraneous and/or supererogatory textbooks.

In short, this PASSBOOK®, used directedly, should be an important factor in helping you to pass your test.

CERTIFIED NURSE EXAMINATION SERIES

NURSING EXAMINATION RESOURCES

A variety of tests and programs are available through a number of organizations that will aid and help prepare candidates for nursing certification:

AMERICAN NURSES CREDENTIALING CENTER (ANCC)

The American Nurses Credentialing Center (ANCC) is a subsidiary of the American Nurses' Association (ANA), and the largest nursing credentialing organization in the United States. The ANCC Commission on Certification offers approximately 40 examinations including advanced practice specialties for nurse practitioners and clinical nurse specialists.

Certification is a most important way for you to show that you are among the best in your field -- an extra step for you and your career, a step *beyond* state licensing. It gives you recognition and status on a *national* basis.

ANCC certification exams are offered twice a year in May and October in paper-and-pencil format, and throughout the year as computer-based exams. All exams are multiple choice and cover knowledge, understanding and application of professional nursing practice and theory. The time allotted for both the paper-and-pencil and computer certification exams is 3 hours and 30 minutes.

Each exam is developed in cooperation with an individual Content Expert Panel (CEP) composed of experts representing specific areas of certification. These panels analyze the professional skills and abilities required and then define which content should be covered and how strongly emphasized. Test questions are written by certified nurses in their discipline and reviewed by the ANCC to ensure validity and quality.

Exams are scored on a scale, and will be reported as either "Pass" or "Fail." Those who fail the exam will receive diagnostic information for each area of the test. There is a minimum 90-day waiting period from the date of the failed exam for those looking to retake it. For those who pass the exam, a certificate, official identification card and pin will be sent. Certification is valid for five years.

For further information and application for admission to candidacy for certification, write to:
American Nurses Credentialing Center
8515 Georgia Ave., Suite 400
Silver Spring, MD 20910-3492

You can also contact the ANCC and receive further details regarding certification exams and registration by visiting its home on the Internet -- www.nursecredentialing.org -- or by phone (1-800-284-CERT). Test Content Outlines (TCO) for each exam can also be found on the ANCC website, detailing the format and content breakdown of the test as well as the content areas the examinee should be prepared for.

NATIONAL CERTIFICATION CORPORATION

NCC CERTIFICATION

NCC – the National Certification Corporation for the Obstetric, Gynecologic and Neonatal Nursing specialties – is an independent certification organization. NCC was established in 1975 as a non-profit corporation for the purpose of sponsoring a volunteer certification program.

BENEFITS OF CERTIFICATION

Certification serves as an added credential to attest to attainment of special knowledge beyond the basic nursing degree. Certification serves to maintain and promote quality nursing care by providing a mechanism to nurses to demonstrate their special knowledge in a specific nursing area.

Promotion of quality care through certification benefits not only the individual nurse and the profession of nursing, but the public as well. Certification documents to employers, professional colleagues and health team members that special knowledge has been achieved, provides for expanded career opportunities and advancement within the specialty of OGN nursing, and elevates the standards of the obstetric, gynecologic and neonatal nursing practice.

Certification granted by NCC is pursuant to a voluntary procedure intended solely to test for special knowledge.

NCC does not purport to license, to confer a right or privilege upon, nor otherwise to define qualifications of any person for nursing practice.

The significance of certification in any jurisdiction or institution is the responsibility of the candidate to determine. The candidate should contact the appropriate state board of nursing or institution.

EXAMINATION DEVELOPMENT

NCC selects educators and practitioners in both nursing and medicine who possess expertise in the specialty areas within the obstetric, gynecologic and neonatal nursing and related fields to serve on the test committees. Responsibilities of the test committees include coordination of overall development of certification examinations and development of materials to assist candidates to assess readiness to participate in the certification process.

EXAMINATION DESCRIPTION

Each of the examinations consists of 200 multiple-choice questions. Two forms of each examination are often given to provide the opportunity to perform statistical procedures which ensure added reliability to the total examination process. The examinations are offered only in English and are designed to test special knowledge.

The examinations are given once each in the morning and afternoon, Monday through Friday, at more than 100 test centers. Four hours are allotted for completion of the examination.

THE CERTIFICATION PROCESS

1. Applicants must complete and file a certification application and appropriate documentation and fees
2. An acknowledgment postcard is sent to each applicant when NCC receives the application
3. Eligibility to participate is determined
4. Applicant is notified of eligibility status and eligible candidate receives a Candidate Guide to NCC Certification (4 to 6 weeks from receipt of application)
5. Candidates will schedule their own appointment for an examination time and location, and must take the exam within a 90-day period from notification of eligibility
6. Test administration occurs
7. Examinations are scored and analyzed
8. Candidates receive score reports upon completion of computerized testing (not paper testing)
9. Candidates are notified of certification status, receive information about certification maintenance and are later issued formal certificates

REVIEW COURSES AND NCC

NCC does not sponsor or endorse any review courses or materials for the certification examinations, because to do so would be a conflict of interest.

NCC is not affiliated with and does not provide input or information for any review courses or materials that other organizations may offer.

NCC views certification as an evaluative process. Eligibility criteria have been established to identify a minimum level of preparation for the exams.

CANDIDATE GUIDE TO NCC CERTIFICATION

Each candidate determined eligible to participate in the NCC certification process will be sent a Guide to NCC Certification. These guides can also be found online at the NCC website (www.nccnet.org). The Candidate Guides contain:

- General policies and procedures about the certification process
- Competency Statements that serve as a role description for the specialty nurse
- Expanded examination content outline
- Bibliography of references
- Sample questions to familiarize candidates with examination format (*These questions are not representative of exam content or difficulty level)

The Candidate Guide is not provided as study material, but to assist candidates in evaluating their own nursing practice as they prepare for the certification examination through identification of potential areas of strength and weakness.

SCORING OF EXAMINATIONS

Passing scores are determined based on a criterion-referenced system. Criterion passing scores are established by the NCC Board of Directors in conjunction with the NCC Test Committees using standard psychometric procedures.

Each question is statistically analyzed and evaluated with psychometric consultation, and scores are computed based on this evaluation.

Candidates who take the computerized form of the certification exam will receive their score reports upon completion of the exam. Those who take the paper/pencil exam will not receive their score reports for several weeks after administration.

NOTIFICATION AND AWARDING OF CERTIFICATION

Each candidate is notified of the success or failure to achieve certification. Successful candidates receive a formal certificate and will be able to use the initial RNC (Registered Nurse Certified) to indicate certification status.

Certification is awarded for a period of three years. Initial certification is effective from the date of notification to December 31 of the third full calendar year following notification. Subsequent periods of certification are subject to policies of the Certification Maintenance Program.

CERTIFICATION MAINTENANCE

The NCC Certification Maintenance Program allows the certified nurse to maintain NCC certification status.

Certification status must be maintained on an ongoing basis every three years through demonstration of approved continuing education or reexamination. Certification that is not maintained through the Certification Maintenance Program may only be regained by reexamination.

Specific information about the Certification Maintenance Program is provided to successful certification candidates and may also be obtained by contacting the NCC website (www.nccnet.org).

GENERAL POLICIES

All required practice experience/employment must have occurred while the applicant is/was a U.S. or Canadian RN. Graduate Nurse or Interim Permit status is acceptable, but must be indicated separately on the application form in addition to original licensure information.

NCC defines employment as practice in any of the following settings: direct patient care, educational institutions, administration or research.

When meeting educational requirements, all coursework, including that not directly related to specialty areas, thesis work and/or other program requirements must be completed at the time the application is filed.

It is the policy of NCC that no individual shall be excluded from the opportunity to participate in the NCC certification program on the basis of race, national origin, religion, sex, age or handicap.

All applications received are subject to the nonrefundable application fee ($250 paper/pencil; $300 computer).

Incomplete applications or applications submitted without appropriate fees will be returned and subject to all policies, fees and deadlines.

Applicants determined eligible (whether the candidate has been notified or not) and withdrawn will be subject to stated refund policies.

All NCC policies and requirements are subject to change without notice.

RETEST POLICIES

The NCC does not limit the number of times a candidate may retake the NCC Certification Examinations. Unsuccessful candidates who wish to be retested must reapply, submit all applicable fees and documentation, and re-establish eligibility.

Eligibility: All eligibility criteria of practice experience and/or educational preparation must be met by the time of application. It is the candidate's decision to choose the appropriate examination, based on the content outline, the individual's practice experience and NCC eligibility criteria.

Forms: All required forms must be submitted, and must include all requested information. If the forms are missing information, your application will be returned or you may be found ineligible to sit for the exam. Be sure the RN licensure information is completed. Be sure your documentation is signed by your supervisor or program director, with his/her title indicated, and the date the form is signed. Review your forms before you submit them.

Fees and Refunds: The proper fee must be submitted with your application or it will be returned.

For a current exam catalog containing current fees, terms, filing deadlines and exam dates, contact the NCC at www.nccnet.org, call (312) 951-0207 or fax at (312) 951-9475.

National Certification Corporation
PO Box 11082
Chicago, IL 60611-0082

CENTER FOR CERTIFICATION PREPARATION AND REVIEW

The Center for Certification Preparation and Review (CCPR) provides practice examinations developed by nurses and is intended to familiarize candidates with the content and feel of the real test. The CCPR practice examination identifies content areas of strength and weakness, provides examples of the type and format of questions that will appear on the examination, as well as information on how to focus additional study efforts.

The CCPR program consists of: study strategies, competency statements, content outline, 160-item examination, answer key and sample answer sheet, performance assessment grid, rationales for answers and cited references. Exams are available for inpatient obstetric, maternal newborn, neonatal intensive care and low-risk neonatal nursing, as well as neonatal nurse practitioner and women's health care nurse practitioner.

More information on ordering these practice exams can be found at www.ccprnet.org.

The National Certification Corporation (NCC), a not-for-profit organization that provides a national credentialing program for nurses, physicians and other licensed health care personnel, offers candidate guides for each of the NCC examinations. These candidate guides contain competency statements, detailed test outlines, sample questions, list of book/periodical references and all NCC policies related to the test administration process.

NCC guides are available in the following areas: inpatient obstetric, low-risk neonatal, maternal newborn and neonatal intensive care nursing, as well as neonatal nurse practitioner, telephone nursing practice, women's health care nurse practitioner, electronic fetal monitoring subspecialty examination, and menopause clinician. These guides, in addition to other information regarding testing, NCC publications and links to other organizations, are available online at www.nccnet.org.

RESOURCES FOR PRE-ADMISSION AND ACHIEVEMENT TESTS IN RN AND PN PROGRAMS

The National League for Nursing (NLN) offers a wide variety of examinations designed to aid students looking to further their education in the field of nursing. NLN pre-admission exams are reliable and valid predictors of student success in nursing programs, and NLN achievement tests allow educators to evaluate course or program objectives and to compare student performance to a national sample. The NLN also provides Diagnostic Readiness Tests, Critical Thinking and Comprehensive Nursing Achievement Exams and Acceleration Challenge Exams.

NLN exams can be ordered in paper form or e-mailed directly to you as online tests. The RN program includes tests in: basic nursing care, nursing care of children, maternity and child health nursing, nursing care of adults, psychiatric mental health and pharmacology in clinical nursing, baccalaureate achievement, physical assessment, community health nursing, comprehensive psychiatric nursing, heath and illness, anatomy and physiology, and microbiology.

NLN achievement tests also cover a PN program, which includes exams in: PN fundamentals, maternity infant, child health and adult health nursing, as well as mental health concepts and PN pharmacology.

NLN Pre-NCLEX Readiness Tests serve as practice and review for the NCLEX. Comprehensive Nursing Achievement, Critical Thinking and Diagnostic Readiness Tests are complementary to one another and help students prepare for nursing practice and to pass the NCLEX.

For in-depth information about the types of tests available, ordering, and additional NLN publications, including the NLN test catalog (available for download), visit www.nln.org.

HOW TO TAKE A TEST

You have studied long, hard and conscientiously.

With your official admission card in hand, and your heart pounding, you have been admitted to the examination room.

You note that there are several hundred other applicants in the examination room waiting to take the same test.

They all appear to be equally well prepared.

You know that nothing but your best effort will suffice. The "moment of truth" is at hand: you now have to demonstrate objectively, in writing, your knowledge of content and your understanding of subject matter.

You are fighting the most important battle of your life—to pass and/or score high on an examination which will determine your career and provide the economic basis for your livelihood.

What extra, special things should you know and should you do in taking the examination?

I. YOU MUST PASS AN EXAMINATION

A. WHAT EVERY CANDIDATE SHOULD KNOW
   Examination applicants often ask us for help in preparing for the written test. What can I study in advance? What kinds of questions will be asked? How will the test be given? How will the papers be graded?

B. HOW ARE EXAMS DEVELOPED?
   Examinations are carefully written by trained technicians who are specialists in the field known as "psychological measurement," in consultation with recognized authorities in the field of work that the test will cover. These experts recommend the subject matter areas or skills to be tested; only those knowledges or skills important to your success on the job are included. The most reliable books and source materials available are used as references. Together, the experts and technicians judge the difficulty level of the questions.
   Test technicians know how to phrase questions so that the problem is clearly stated. Their ethics do not permit "trick" or "catch" questions. Questions may have been tried out on sample groups, or subjected to statistical analysis, to determine their usefulness.
   Written tests are often used in combination with performance tests, ratings of training and experience, and oral interviews. All of these measures combine to form the best-known means of finding the right person for the right job.

II. HOW TO PASS THE WRITTEN TEST

A. BASIC STEPS

1) Study the announcement

How, then, can you know what subjects to study? Our best answer is: "Learn as much as possible about the class of positions for which you've applied." The exam will test the knowledge, skills and abilities needed to do the work.

Your most valuable source of information about the position you want is the official exam announcement. This announcement lists the training and experience qualifications. Check these standards and apply only if you come reasonably close to meeting them. Many jurisdictions preview the written test in the exam announcement by including a section called "Knowledge and Abilities Required," "Scope of the Examination," or some similar heading. Here you will find out specifically what fields will be tested.

2) Choose appropriate study materials

If the position for which you are applying is technical or advanced, you will read more advanced, specialized material. If you are already familiar with the basic principles of your field, elementary textbooks would waste your time. Concentrate on advanced textbooks and technical periodicals. Think through the concepts and review difficult problems in your field.

These are all general sources. You can get more ideas on your own initiative, following these leads. For example, training manuals and publications of the government agency which employs workers in your field can be useful, particularly for technical and professional positions. A letter or visit to the government department involved may result in more specific study suggestions, and certainly will provide you with a more definite idea of the exact nature of the position you are seeking.

3) Study this book!

III. KINDS OF TESTS

Tests are used for purposes other than measuring knowledge and ability to perform specified duties. For some positions, it is equally important to test ability to make adjustments to new situations or to profit from training. In others, basic mental abilities not dependent on information are essential. Questions which test these things may not appear as pertinent to the duties of the position as those which test for knowledge and information. Yet they are often highly important parts of a fair examination. For very general questions, it is almost impossible to help you direct your study efforts. What we can do is to point out some of the more common of these general abilities needed in public service positions and describe some typical questions.

1) General information

Broad, general information has been found useful for predicting job success in some kinds of work. This is tested in a variety of ways, from vocabulary lists to questions about current events. Basic background in some field of work, such as sociology or economics, may be sampled in a group of questions. Often these are principles which have become familiar to most persons through exposure rather than through formal training. It is difficult to advise you how to study for these questions; being alert to the world around you is our best suggestion.

2) Verbal ability

An example of an ability needed in many positions is verbal or language ability. Verbal ability is, in brief, the ability to use and understand words. Vocabulary and grammar tests are typical measures of this ability. Reading comprehension or paragraph interpretation questions are common in many kinds of civil service tests. You are given a paragraph of written material and asked to find its central meaning.

IV. KINDS OF QUESTIONS

1. Multiple-choice Questions

Most popular of the short-answer questions is the "multiple choice" or "best answer" question. It can be used, for example, to test for factual knowledge, ability to solve problems or judgment in meeting situations found at work.

A multiple-choice question is normally one of three types:
- It can begin with an incomplete statement followed by several possible endings. You are to find the one ending which best completes the statement, although some of the others may not be entirely wrong.
- It can also be a complete statement in the form of a question which is answered by choosing one of the statements listed.
- It can be in the form of a problem – again you select the best answer.

Here is an example of a multiple-choice question with a discussion which should give you some clues as to the method for choosing the right answer:

When an employee has a complaint about his assignment, the action which will best help him overcome his difficulty is to
- A. discuss his difficulty with his coworkers
- B. take the problem to the head of the organization
- C. take the problem to the person who gave him the assignment
- D. say nothing to anyone about his complaint

In answering this question, you should study each of the choices to find which is best. Consider choice "A" – Certainly an employee may discuss his complaint with fellow employees, but no change or improvement can result, and the complaint remains unresolved. Choice "B" is a poor choice since the head of the organization probably does not know what assignment you have been given, and taking your problem to him is known as "going over the head" of the supervisor. The supervisor, or person who made the assignment, is the person who can clarify it or correct any injustice. Choice "C" is, therefore, correct. To say nothing, as in choice "D," is unwise. Supervisors have and interest in knowing the problems employees are facing, and the employee is seeking a solution to his problem.

2. True/False

3. Matching Questions

Matching an answer from a column of choices within another column.

V. RECORDING YOUR ANSWERS

Computer terminals are used more and more today for many different kinds of exams.

For an examination with very few applicants, you may be told to record your answers in the test booklet itself. Separate answer sheets are much more common. If this separate answer sheet is to be scored by machine – and this is often the case – it is highly important that you mark your answers correctly in order to get credit.

VI. BEFORE THE TEST

YOUR PHYSICAL CONDITION IS IMPORTANT

If you are not well, you can't do your best work on tests. If you are half asleep, you can't do your best either. Here are some tips:

1) Get about the same amount of sleep you usually get. Don't stay up all night before the test, either partying or worrying—DON'T DO IT!
2) If you wear glasses, be sure to wear them when you go to take the test. This goes for hearing aids, too.
3) If you have any physical problems that may keep you from doing your best, be sure to tell the person giving the test. If you are sick or in poor health, you relay cannot do your best on any test. You can always come back and take the test some other time.

Common sense will help you find procedures to follow to get ready for an examination. Too many of us, however, overlook these sensible measures. Indeed, nervousness and fatigue have been found to be the most serious reasons why applicants fail to do their best on civil service tests. Here is a list of reminders:

- Begin your preparation early – Don't wait until the last minute to go scurrying around for books and materials or to find out what the position is all about.
- Prepare continuously – An hour a night for a week is better than an all-night cram session. This has been definitely established. What is more, a night a week for a month will return better dividends than crowding your study into a shorter period of time.
- Locate the place of the exam – You have been sent a notice telling you when and where to report for the examination. If the location is in a different town or otherwise unfamiliar to you, it would be well to inquire the best route and learn something about the building.
- Relax the night before the test – Allow your mind to rest. Do not study at all that night. Plan some mild recreation or diversion; then go to bed early and get a good night's sleep.
- Get up early enough to make a leisurely trip to the place for the test – This way unforeseen events, traffic snarls, unfamiliar buildings, etc. will not upset you.
- Dress comfortably – A written test is not a fashion show. You will be known by number and not by name, so wear something comfortable.
- Leave excess paraphernalia at home – Shopping bags and odd bundles will get in your way. You need bring only the items mentioned in the official notice you received; usually everything you need is provided. Do not bring reference books to the exam. They will only confuse those last minutes and be taken away from you when in the test room.

- Arrive somewhat ahead of time – If because of transportation schedules you must get there very early, bring a newspaper or magazine to take your mind off yourself while waiting.
- Locate the examination room – When you have found the proper room, you will be directed to the seat or part of the room where you will sit. Sometimes you are given a sheet of instructions to read while you are waiting. Do not fill out any forms until you are told to do so; just read them and be prepared.
- Relax and prepare to listen to the instructions
- If you have any physical problem that may keep you from doing your best, be sure to tell the test administrator. If you are sick or in poor health, you really cannot do your best on the exam. You can come back and take the test some other time.

VII. AT THE TEST

The day of the test is here and you have the test booklet in your hand. The temptation to get going is very strong. Caution! There is more to success than knowing the right answers. You must know how to identify your papers and understand variations in the type of short-answer question used in this particular examination. Follow these suggestions for maximum results from your efforts:

1) Cooperate with the monitor

The test administrator has a duty to create a situation in which you can be as much at ease as possible. He will give instructions, tell you when to begin, check to see that you are marking your answer sheet correctly, and so on. He is not there to guard you, although he will see that your competitors do not take unfair advantage. He wants to help you do your best.

2) Listen to all instructions

Don't jump the gun! Wait until you understand all directions. In most civil service tests you get more time than you need to answer the questions. So don't be in a hurry. Read each word of instructions until you clearly understand the meaning. Study the examples, listen to all announcements and follow directions. Ask questions if you do not understand what to do.

3) Identify your papers

Civil service exams are usually identified by number only. You will be assigned a number; you must not put your name on your test papers. Be sure to copy your number correctly. Since more than one exam may be given, copy your exact examination title.

4) Plan your time

Unless you are told that a test is a "speed" or "rate of work" test, speed itself is usually not important. Time enough to answer all the questions will be provided, but this does not mean that you have all day. An overall time limit has been set. Divide the total time (in minutes) by the number of questions to determine the approximate time you have for each question.

5) Do not linger over difficult questions

If you come across a difficult question, mark it with a paper clip (useful to have along) and come back to it when you have been through the booklet. One caution if you do this – be sure to skip a number on your answer sheet as well. Check often to be sure that you have not lost your place and that you are marking in the row numbered the same as the question you are answering.

6) Read the questions

Be sure you know what the question asks! Many capable people are unsuccessful because they failed to read the questions correctly.

7) Answer all questions

Unless you have been instructed that a penalty will be deducted for incorrect answers, it is better to guess than to omit a question.

8) Speed tests

It is often better NOT to guess on speed tests. It has been found that on timed tests people are tempted to spend the last few seconds before time is called in marking answers at random – without even reading them – in the hope of picking up a few extra points. To discourage this practice, the instructions may warn you that your score will be "corrected" for guessing. That is, a penalty will be applied. The incorrect answers will be deducted from the correct ones, or some other penalty formula will be used.

9) Review your answers

If you finish before time is called, go back to the questions you guessed or omitted to give them further thought. Review other answers if you have time.

10) Return your test materials

If you are ready to leave before others have finished or time is called, take ALL your materials to the monitor and leave quietly. Never take any test material with you. The monitor can discover whose papers are not complete, and taking a test booklet may be grounds for disqualification.

VIII. EXAMINATION TECHNIQUES

1) Read the general instructions carefully. These are usually printed on the first page of the exam booklet. As a rule, these instructions refer to the timing of the examination; the fact that you should not start work until the signal and must stop work at a signal, etc. If there are any special instructions, such as a choice of questions to be answered, make sure that you note this instruction carefully.

2) When you are ready to start work on the examination, that is as soon as the signal has been given, read the instructions to each question booklet, underline any key words or phrases, such as least, best, outline, describe and the like. In this way you will tend to answer as requested rather than discover on reviewing your paper that you listed without describing, that you selected the worst choice rather than the best choice, etc.

3) If the examination is of the objective or multiple-choice type – that is, each question will also give a series of possible answers: A, B, C or D, and you are called upon to select the best answer and write the letter next to that answer on your answer paper – it is advisable to start answering each question in turn. There may be anywhere from 50 to 100 such questions in the three or four hours allotted and you can see how much time would be taken if you read through all the questions before beginning to answer any. Furthermore, if you

come across a question or group of questions which you know would be difficult to answer, it would undoubtedly affect your handling of all the other questions.

4) If the examination is of the essay type and contains but a few questions, it is a moot point as to whether you should read all the questions before starting to answer any one. Of course, if you are given a choice – say five out of seven and the like – then it is essential to read all the questions so you can eliminate the two that are most difficult. If, however, you are asked to answer all the questions, there may be danger in trying to answer the easiest one first because you may find that you will spend too much time on it. The best technique is to answer the first question, then proceed to the second, etc.

5) Time your answers. Before the exam begins, write down the time it started, then add the time allowed for the examination and write down the time it must be completed, then divide the time available somewhat as follows:
    - If 3-1/2 hours are allowed, that would be 210 minutes. If you have 80 objective-type questions, that would be an average of 2-1/2 minutes per question. Allow yourself no more than 2 minutes per question, or a total of 160 minutes, which will permit about 50 minutes to review.
    - If for the time allotment of 210 minutes there are 7 essay questions to answer, that would average about 30 minutes a question. Give yourself only 25 minutes per question so that you have about 35 minutes to review.

6) The most important instruction is to read each question and make sure you know what is wanted. The second most important instruction is to time yourself properly so that you answer every question. The third most important instruction is to answer every question. Guess if you have to but include something for each question. Remember that you will receive no credit for a blank and will probably receive some credit if you write something in answer to an essay question. If you guess a letter – say "B" for a multiple-choice question – you may have guessed right. If you leave a blank as an answer to a multiple-choice question, the examiners may respect your feelings but it will not add a point to your score. Some exams may penalize you for wrong answers, so in such cases only, you may not want to guess unless you have some basis for your answer.

7) Suggestions
    a. Objective-type questions
        1. Examine the question booklet for proper sequence of pages and questions
        2. Read all instructions carefully
        3. Skip any question which seems too difficult; return to it after all other questions have been answered
        4. Apportion your time properly; do not spend too much time on any single question or group of questions
        5. Note and underline key words – all, most, fewest, least, best, worst, same, opposite, etc.
        6. Pay particular attention to negatives
        7. Note unusual option, e.g., unduly long, short, complex, different or similar in content to the body of the question
        8. Observe the use of "hedging" words – probably, may, most likely, etc.

9. Make sure that your answer is put next to the same number as the question
10. Do not second-guess unless you have good reason to believe the second answer is definitely more correct
11. Cross out original answer if you decide another answer is more accurate; do not erase until you are ready to hand your paper in
12. Answer all questions; guess unless instructed otherwise
13. Leave time for review

b. Essay questions
 1. Read each question carefully
 2. Determine exactly what is wanted. Underline key words or phrases.
 3. Decide on outline or paragraph answer
 4. Include many different points and elements unless asked to develop any one or two points or elements
 5. Show impartiality by giving pros and cons unless directed to select one side only
 6. Make and write down any assumptions you find necessary to answer the questions
 7. Watch your English, grammar, punctuation and choice of words
 8. Time your answers; don't crowd material

8) Answering the essay question

Most essay questions can be answered by framing the specific response around several key words or ideas. Here are a few such key words or ideas:

M's: manpower, materials, methods, money, management
P's: purpose, program, policy, plan, procedure, practice, problems, pitfalls, personnel, public relations

a. Six basic steps in handling problems:
 1. Preliminary plan and background development
 2. Collect information, data and facts
 3. Analyze and interpret information, data and facts
 4. Analyze and develop solutions as well as make recommendations
 5. Prepare report and sell recommendations
 6. Install recommendations and follow up effectiveness

b. Pitfalls to avoid
 1. Taking things for granted – A statement of the situation does not necessarily imply that each of the elements is necessarily true; for example, a complaint may be invalid and biased so that all that can be taken for granted is that a complaint has been registered
 2. Considering only one side of a situation – Wherever possible, indicate several alternatives and then point out the reasons you selected the best one
 3. Failing to indicate follow up – Whenever your answer indicates action on your part, make certain that you will take proper follow-up action to see how successful your recommendations, procedures or actions turn out to be
 4. Taking too long in answering any single question – Remember to time your answers properly

EXAMINATION SECTION

EXAMINATION SECTION
TEST 1

DIRECTIONS: Each question or incomplete statement is followed by several suggested answers or completions. Select the one that BEST answers the question or completes the statement. *PRINT THE LETTER OF THE CORRECT ANSWER IN THE SPACE AT THE RIGHT.*

1. The abbreviation *EEG* refers to a(n)

    A. examination of the eyes and ears
    B. inflammatory disease of the urinogenital tract
    C. disease of the esophageal structure
    D. examination of the brain

    1._____

2. The complete destruction of all forms of living microorganisms is called

    A. decontamination
    B. sterilization
    C. fumigation
    D. germination

    2._____

3. A rectal thermometer differs from other fever thermometers in that it has a

    A. longer stem
    B. thinner stem
    C. stubby bulb at one end
    D. slender bulb at one end

    3._____

4. The one of the following pieces of equipment which is USUALLY used together with a sphygmometer is a

    A. stethoscope
    B. watch
    C. fever thermometer
    D. hypodermic syringe

    4._____

5. A curette is a

    A. healing drug
    B. curved scalpel
    C. long hypodermic needle
    D. scraping instrument

    5._____

6. The otoscope is used to examine the patient's

    A. eyes   B. ears   C. mouth   D. lungs

    6._____

7. A catheter is used

    A. to close wounds
    B. for withdrawing fluid from a body cavity
    C. to remove cataracts
    D. as a cathartic

    7._____

8. Of the following pieces of equipment, the one that is required for making a scratch test is a

    A. needle   B. scalpel   C. capillary tube   D. tourniquet

    8._____

9. A hemostat is an instrument which is used to

    A. hold a sterile needle
    B. clamp off a blood vessel
    C. regulate the temperature of a sterilizer
    D. measure oxygen intake

    9._____

1

10. Of the following medical supplies, the one that MUST be stored in a tightly sealed bottle is

    A. sodium fluoride
    B. alum
    C. oil of cloves
    D. aromatic spirits of ammonia

11. A person who has been exposed to an infectious disease is called

    A. a contact
    B. an incubator
    C. diseased
    D. infected

12. A myocardial infarct would occur in the

    A. heart   B. kidneys   C. lungs   D. spleen

13. The abbreviations *WBC* and *RBC* refer to the results of tests of the

    A. basal metabolism
    B. blood
    C. blood pressure
    D. bony structure

14. When a person's blood pressure is noted as 120/80, it means that his

    A. pulse blood pressure is 120
    B. pulse blood pressure is 80
    C. systolic blood pressure is 120
    D. systolic blood pressure is 80

15. The anatomical structure that contains the tonsils and adenoids is the

    A. pharynx   B. larynx   C. trachea   D. sinuses

16. An abscess can BEST be described as a

    A. loss of sensation
    B. painful tooth
    C. ruptured membrane
    D. localized formation of pus

17. Nephritis is a disease affecting the

    A. gall bladder
    B. larynx
    C. kidney
    D. large intestine

18. Hemoglobin is contained in the

    A. white blood cells
    B. lymph fluids
    C. platelets
    D. red blood cells

19. Bile is a body fluid that is MOST directly concerned with

    A. digestion
    B. excretion
    C. reproduction
    D. metabolism

20. Of the following bones, the one which is located BELOW the waist is the

    A. sternum   B. clavicle   C. tibia   D. humerus

21. The one of the following which is NOT part of the digestive canal is the   21._____
    A. esophagus   B. larynx   C. duodenum   D. colon

22. The thyroid and the pituitary are part of the _____ system.   22._____
    A. digestive   B. endocrine
    C. respiratory   D. excretory

23. The one of the following which would be included in a *GU* examination is the   23._____
    A. rectum   B. trachea   C. kidneys   D. pancreas

24. Of the following, the one which would be included in the x-ray examination known as a *GI series* is the   24._____
    A. colon   B. skull   C. lungs   D. uterus

25. A person who, while not ill himself, may transmit a disease to another person is known as a(n)   25._____
    A. breeder   B. incubator
    C. carrier   D. inhibitor

KEY (CORRECT ANSWERS)

1.	D	11.	A
2.	C	12.	A
3.	C	13.	B
4.	A	14.	C
5.	D	15.	A
6.	B	16.	D
7.	B	17.	C
8.	A	18.	D
9.	B	19.	A
10.	D	20.	C

21. B
22. B
23. C
24. A
25. C

TEST 2

DIRECTIONS: Each question or incomplete statement is followed by several suggested answers or completions. Select the one that BEST answers the question or completes the statement. *PRINT THE LETTER OF THE CORRECT ANSWER IN THE SPACE AT THE RIGHT.*

1. Thorough washing of the hands for two minutes with soap and warm water will leave the hands 1.____

    A. sterile
    B. aseptic
    C. decontaminated
    D. partially disinfected

2. The one of the following which is BEST for preparing the skin for an injection is 2.____

    A. green soap and water
    B. alcohol
    C. phenol
    D. formalin

3. A fever thermometer should be cleansed after use by washing it with 3.____

    A. soap and cool water
    B. warm water only
    C. soap and hot water
    D. running cold tap water

4. The FIRST step in cleaning an instrument which has fresh blood on it is to 4.____

    A. wash it in hot soapy water
    B. wash it under cool running water
    C. soak it in a boric acid bath
    D. soak it in 70% alcohol

5. If a contaminated nasal speculum cannot be sterilized immediately after use, then the BEST procedure to follow until sterilization is possible is to place it 5.____

    A. under a piece of dry *gauze*
    B. in warm water
    C. in alcohol
    D. in a green soap solution

6. A hypodermic needle should ALWAYS be checked to see whether it has a good sharp point 6.____

    A. when it is being washed
    B. when it is removed from the sterilizer
    C. just before it is sterilized
    D. immediately before an injection

7. Of the following, the LOWEST temperature at which cotton goods will be sterilized if placed in an autoclave for 30 minutes is 7.____

    A. 130° F B. 170° F C. 200° F D. 250° F

8. Of the following procedures, the one which is BEST for sterilizing an ear speculum which is contaminated with wax is to

   A. scrub it with cold soapy water, rinse in ether, and place in boiling water for 20 minutes
   B. soak it in warm water, scrub in cold soapy water, rinse with water, and autoclave at 275° F for 10 minutes
   C. wash it in alcohol, scrub in hot soapy water, rinse with water, and place in boiling water for 20 minutes
   D. wash it in 1% Lysol solution, rinse, and autoclave at 275° F for 15 minutes

9. Assume that clean water accidentally spilled on the outside of a package of cloth-wrapped hypodermic syringes which has been sterilized.
   Of the following, the BEST action to take is to

   A. leave the package to dry in a sunny, clean place
   B. sterilize the package again
   C. remove the wet cloth and wrap the package in a dry sterile cloth
   D. wipe off the package with a clean dry towel and later ask the nurse-in-charge what to do

10. Hypodermic needles should be sterilized by placing them in

    A. boiling water for 5 minutes
    B. an autoclave at 15 lbs. pressure for 15 minutes
    C. oil heated to 220° F for 10 minutes
    D. a 1:40 Lysol solution for 10 minutes

11. A cutting instrument should be sterilized by placing it in

    A. a chemical germicide
    B. an autoclave at 15 lbs. pressure for 20 minutes
    C. boiling water for 20 minutes
    D. a hot air oven at 320° F for 1 hour

12. A fever thermometer used by a patient who has tuberculosis should be washed and then placed in

    A. boiling water for 10 minutes
    B. a hot air oven for 20 minutes
    C. a 1:1000 solution of bichloride of mercury for one minute
    D. an autoclave at 15 lbs. pressure for 15 minutes

13. The MOST reliable method of sterilizing a glass syringe is to place it in

    A. Zephiran chloride 1:1000 solution for 40 minutes
    B. oil heated to 250° F for 12 minutes
    C. boiling water for 20 minutes
    D. an autoclave at 15 lbs. pressure for 20 minutes

14. The insides of sterilizers should be cleaned daily with a mild abrasive PRIMARILY to

   A. remove scale
   B. prevent the growth of bacteria
   C. remove blood and other organic matter
   D. prevent acids from damaging the sterilizer

15. Of the following, the BEST reason for giving a patient a jar in which to bring a urine specimen on his next visit to the clinic is that the

   A. patient may not have a jar at home
   B. patient may bring the specimen in a jar which is too large
   C. patient may bring the specimen in a jar which has not been cleaned properly
   D. jar may be misplaced if it is not a jar in which urine specimens are usually collected

16. Of the following, the MOST important reason why you should remain with a 4-year-old child when his temperature is being taken by mouth is that otherwise the child might

   A. fall off the chair and fracture an arm or leg
   B. break the thermometer while it is in his mouth
   C. remove the thermometer from his mouth and misplace it
   D. leave the examining room and return to his mother

17. The BEST way to take the temperature of an infant is by

   A. feeling his forehead
   B. using an oral thermometer
   C. placing a thermometer under his armpit
   D. using a rectal thermometer

18. When the temperature of an adult is taken rectally, it is LEAST accurate to say that the

   A. temperature reading will be higher than if it were taken orally
   B. thermometer should be lubricated before use
   C. thermometer should be in place for at least ten minutes
   D. temperature reading is likely to be more accurate than if it were taken orally

19. When the temperature of an adult is taken orally, it is LEAST accurate to say that the

   A. thermometer should be washed with alcohol before it is used
   B. thermometer should be taken down below 96° F before it is used
   C. patient's temperature may be taken immediately after he has smoked a cigarette
   D. patient should be inactive just before his temperature is taken

20. The nurse described the test to the patient before bringing him to the examining room for a basal metabolism test. Her action may BEST be described as

   A. *correct;* the patient will be more cooperative if he knows what to expect
   B. *wrong;* the nurse does not know how the test will affect the patient
   C. *correct;* the nurse can judge whether the patient is too upset by this information to take the test
   D. *wrong;* explaining the test beforehand will only make the patient nervous

21. When a patient's sputum test is *positive,* it means that the 21.____
    A. patient's sputum is plentiful
    B. doctor has made an accurate diagnosis
    C. patient has recovered and is now in good health
    D. laboratory reports that the patient's sputum contains certain disease germs

22. A biopsy can BEST be described as a(n) 22.____
    A. pre-cancerous condition   B. examination of tissues
    C. living organism   D. germicidal solution

23. The *scratch* or *patch* test is USUALLY given when testing for 23.____
    A. allergies   B. rheumatic fever
    C. blood poisoning   D. diabetes

24. Gamma globulin is frequently given to children after exposure to and before the appearance of symptoms of 24.____
    A. measles   B. smallpox
    C. tetanus   D. chicken pox

25. Of the following, the one which is NOT a respiratory disease is 25.____
    A. bronchitis   B. pneumonia
    C. nephritis   D. croup

KEY (CORRECT ANSWERS)

1.	D	11.	A
2.	B	12.	C
3.	A	13.	D
4.	B	14.	A
5.	D	15.	C
6.	C	16.	B
7.	D	17.	D
8.	C	18.	C
9.	B	19.	C
10.	B	20.	A

21. D
22. B
23. A
24. A
25. C

TEST 3

DIRECTIONS: Each question or incomplete statement is followed by several suggested answers or completions. Select the one that BEST answers the question or completes the statement. *PRINT THE LETTER OF THE CORRECT ANSWER IN THE SPACE AT THE RIGHT.*

1. A physician who specializes in the treatment of conditions affecting the skin is known as a(n)   1.____

   A. urologist
   B. dermatologist
   C. toxicologist
   D. ophthalmologist

2. The branch of medicine which deals with diseases peculiar to women is   2.____

   A. pathology
   B. orthopedics
   C. neurology
   D. gynecology

3. The branch of medicine which deals with diseases of old age is called   3.____

   A. pediatrics
   B. geriatrics
   C. serology
   D. histology

4. *Petit mal* is a form of   4.____

   A. epilepsy   B. syphilis   C. diabetes   D. malaria

5. Glaucoma is a disease of the   5.____

   A. thyroid gland
   B. liver
   C. bladder
   D. eye

6. A patient who has edema has   6.____

   A. not enough red blood cells
   B. too much water in the body tissues
   C. blood in the urine
   D. a swollen gland

7. The thoracic area of the body is located in the   7.____

   A. abdomen
   B. lower back
   C. chest
   D. neck

8. An electrocardiograph is MOST usually used in the examination of the   8.____

   A. brain
   B. heart
   C. kidney
   D. gall bladder

9. The word *coagulate* means MOST NEARLY to   9.____

   A. bleed excessively
   B. break up
   C. work together
   D. form a clot

10. A stethoscope is used to examine the patient's   10.____

    A. heart
    B. patellar reflex
    C. blood cells
    D. spinal fluid

11. A pelvimeter is MOST usually used in the examination of a patient in the _____ clinic.   11.____

    A. chest   B. cancer   C. prenatal   D. eye

12. Tuberculin may BEST be described as a   12.____

    A. virus infection of the lungs
    B. preparation used in the diagnosis of tuberculosis
    C. sanitarium for tuberculous patients
    D. form of cancer of the lung

13. An autoclave is a(n)   13.____

    A. automatic dispenser of instruments needed for clinic examinations
    B. sterile place for storing clinic supplies until they are needed
    C. apparatus for sterilizing equipment under steam pressure
    D. portable self-operating general anesthesia unit

14. Radiation therapy is   14.____

    A. the recording of electrical impulses of the body on a graph
    B. a study of the effects of radiation fall-out on the human body
    C. a form of treatment used for certain diseases
    D. the filming of internal parts of the body through the use of x-rays

15. Diathermy is the treatment of patients by   15.____

    A. scientific use of baths and mineral waters
    B. insertion of radium into diseased tissues
    C. intravenous feedings of vitamins and minerals
    D. electrical generation of heat in the body tissues

16. The measurement of blood pressure involves two readings, which are known as   16.____

    A. metabolic and diastolic
    B. systolic and diastolic
    C. metabolic and hyperbolic
    D. hyperbolic and systolic

17. The Snellen chart is used in examinations of the   17.____

    A. eyes   B. blood   C. urine   D. bile

18. An enema is MOST generally used to   18.____

    A. induce vomiting
    B. irrigate the stomach
    C. clear the bowels
    D. drain the urinary bladder

19. A bronchoscope is USUALLY used in examinations of the   19.____

    A. kidneys   B. heart   C. stomach   D. lungs

20. The Wassermann test is used to find out whether a patient has

   A. diphtheria B. leukemia
   C. scarlet fever D. syphilis

21. If a boiling water sterilizer is used, the minimum time necessary to sterilize instruments is MOST NEARLY _____ hour(s).

   A. 1/2 B. 1 C. 1 1/2 D. 2

22. To sterilize towels and dry gauze dressings in the health clinic, it is MOST advisable to

   A. dip them in a sterilizing solution
   B. wash them with a strong detergent
   C. boil them in the sterilizer
   D. steam them under pressure

23. Sterilization by use of chemicals rather than by boiling water is indicated when the instrument

   A. is made of soft rubber
   B. has a sharp cutting edge
   C. has pus or blood on it
   D. was used more than 24 hours before sterilization

24. When dusting the furniture in the clinic, it is advisable to use a silicone-treated dustcloth CHIEFLY because the treated cloth will

   A. collect the dust more efficiently
   B. disinfect as well as dust the furniture
   C. not remove the wax from the furniture
   D. make it unnecessary to polish the furniture in the future

25. Assume that the clinic in which you work has issued instructions that all supplies containing poison are to have blue labels with the word *poison* clearly marked on the label, and that these supplies are to be kept in a storage cabinet separate from other supplies. You notice that a bottle with no label is on a shelf in the *poison* storage cabinet.
Of the following, the BEST action for you to take is to

   A. place the unlabeled bottle in the back of the regular storage cabinet
   B. put a blue label on the bottle and write *poison* on the label
   C. ask another public health employee to help you decide if the bottle contains poison
   D. pour the contents of the bottle into the slop sink and destroy the bottle

KEY (CORRECT ANSWERS)

1. B
2. D
3. B
4. A
5. D

6. B
7. C
8. B
9. D
10. A

11. C
12. B
13. C
14. C
15. D

16. B
17. A
18. C
19. D
20. D

21. A
22. D
23. B
24. A
25. D

TEST 4

DIRECTIONS: Each question or incomplete statement is followed by several suggested answers or completions. Select the one that BEST answers the question or completes the statement. *PRINT THE LETTER OF THE CORRECT ANSWER IN THE SPACE AT THE RIGHT.*

1. When storing medical supplies, it is important to remember that liquids should be labeled   1._____

    A. only if the liquids are poisonous and there is the slightest chance that they will not be recognized
    B. whenever there is the slightest chance that they will not be recognized
    C. at all times and discarded if labels have become detached
    D. only in those cases where the liquids will be given to patients

2. When dusting metal counter tops in the clinic, it is BEST to use a clean cloth which is   2._____

    A. medicated   B. wet   C. dry   D. damp

3. Of the following statements concerning a hypodermic syringe, the one that is MOST correct is that a plunger   3._____

    A. used for taking blood specimens can be used with any syringe barrel
    B. can be used for any syringe barrel as long as it goes in easily
    C. can be used only with the syringe barrel that was made for it
    D. must be used with the syringe barrel that was made for it only if it is to be used for injections

4. The one of the following which should NOT be done when using a thermometer is to   4._____

    A. shake down the thermometer to 95° F before taking the patient's temperature
    B. ask the patient to keep his lips closed when taking the temperature orally
    C. wash the thermometer in hot soapy water after use
    D. keep the thermometer in a container of alcohol when not in use

5. The temperature of an adult when taken by rectum is USUALLY   5._____

    A. *higher* than if taken either by mouth or under the armpit
    B. *higher* than if taken by mouth and lower than if taken under the armpit
    C. *lower* than if taken either by mouth or under the armpit
    D. *lower* than if taken by mouth and higher than if taken under the armpit

6. Of the following tests, the one which is associated with tuberculosis is the _____ test.   6._____

    A. Schick   B. Mantoux   C. Dick   D. Kahn

7. A needle that has been used to draw blood should be rinsed immediately after use in   7._____

    A. a disinfectant solution   B. hot water
    C. cold water   D. hot, soapy water

8. Of the following, the statement that is MOST correct is that a hypodermic needle should be checked for burrs, hooks, and sharpness

   A. once a week
   B. before it is sterilized
   C. after it has been sterilized
   D. after it has been used three or four times

9. The MOST accurate of the following statements is that when a syringe and needle are being sterilized by boiling, the

   A. plunger must be completely out of the barrel
   B. needle should be left attached to the barrel as when in use
   C. plunger may be completely inside the barrel
   D. needle should be boiled at least twice as long as the syringe

10. Of the following, the MOST important reason for washing an instrument in hot, soapy water is to

    A. sterilize the instrument
    B. destroy germs by heat
    C. destroy germs by coagulation
    D. remove foreign matter and bacteria

11. Assume that a hypodermic needle which is to be used for injection is accidentally brushed at the tip by your hand. Of the following, the action which should be taken before this needle is used is that it be

    A. washed under the hot water tap
    B. wiped with a sterile piece of gauze
    C. washed in hot, soapy water, then rinsed in sterile water
    D. boiled for ten minutes

12. The CORRECT way to sterilize a scalpel is to

    A. place it in a chemical germicide
    B. boil it for 10 minutes
    C. put it in the autoclave
    D. pass it through a bright flame

13. Assume that a tray of instruments has been accidentally left uncovered for five minutes after it had been sterilized.
    Of the following, the action you should take to ensure that the instruments are sterile for use is to

    A. dip them in boiling water
    B. boil them for 10 minutes
    C. replace the cover on the tray
    D. wipe each instrument with sterile gauze

14. An intramuscular injection is MOST likely to be used in the administration of

    A. smallpox vaccine   B. streptomycin
    C. glucose   D. blood

15. The one of the following which is NOT a normal element of blood is 15.____

    A. hemoglobin B. a leucocyte
    C. marrow D. a platelet

16. Of the following statements regarding the Salk vaccine, the MOST accurate one is that it 16.____

    A. immunizes children and adults against paralytic poliomyelit is
    B. is a test to determine the presence of poliomyelitis virus in the blood
    C. is a test to determine whether a child is immune to poliomyelitis
    D. is used in the treatment of patients suffering from paralytic poliomyelitis

17. The GREATEST success in the treatment of cancer has been in cancer of the 17.____

    A. blood B. stomach C. liver D. skin

18. An autopsy is a(n) 18.____

    A. type of blood test
    B. examination of tissue removed from a living organism
    C. examination of a human body after death
    D. test to determine the acidity of body fluids

19. The word *vascular* is MOST closely associated with 19.____

    A. the circulatory system B. respiration
    C. digestion D. the nervous system

20. The word *diagnosis* means MOST NEARLY 20.____

    A. preparation of a diagram
    B. determination of an illness
    C. medical examination of a patient
    D. written prescription

21. A tendon connects 21.____

    A. bone to bone B. muscle to bone
    C. muscle to muscle D. muscle to ligament

22. Blood takes on oxygen as it passes through the 22.____

    A. liver B. heart C. spleen D. lungs

23. The fatty substance in the blood which is deposited in the artery walls and which is believed to cause hardening of the arteries is called 23.____

    A. amino acid B. phenol
    C. cholesterol D. pectin

24. The digestive canal includes the 24.____

    A. stomach, small intestine, large intestine, and rectum
    B. stomach, larynx, large intestine, and rectum
    C. trachea, small intestine, large intestine, and rectum
    D. stomach, small intestine, large intestine, and abdominal cavity

25. When giving artificial respiration, it should be kept in mind that air is drawn into the lungs by the   25._____

    A. expansion of the chest cavity
    B. contraction of the chest cavity
    C. expansion of the lungs
    D. contraction of the lungs

KEY (CORRECT ANSWERS)

1.	C	11.	D
2.	D	12.	A
3.	C	13.	B
4.	C	14.	B
5.	A	15.	C
6.	B	16.	A
7.	C	17.	D
8.	B	18.	C
9.	A	19.	A
10.	D	20.	B

21. B
22. D
23. C
24. A
25. A

EXAMINATION SECTION
TEST 1

DIRECTIONS: Each question or incomplete statement is followed by several suggested answers or completions. Select the one that BEST answers the question or completes the statement. *PRINT THE LETTER OF THE CORRECT ANSWER IN THE SPACE AT THE RIGHT.*

1. A relationship in which a patient becomes dependent on the nurse   1._____

    A. is always unprofessional
    B. is inevitably "bad" for the patient
    C. may be necessary temporarily
    D. impedes learning

2. Anxiety is the CHIEF characteristic of the   2._____

    A. immature personality
    B. psychoneurotic disorder
    C. involutional psychotic reaction
    D. mentally retarded adolescent

3. The mode of psychological adjustment known as regression can BEST be described as   3._____

    A. refusing to think of unpleasant situations
    B. changing to a type of behavior which is characteristic of an earlier period in life
    C. reverting to actions characteristic of an historically early or primitive code of behavior
    D. hostility towards persons or objects that prove frustrating

4. The CHIEF danger in the employment of escape mechanisms as a form of adjustment is that they   4._____

    A. do more harm than good
    B. are socially undesirable
    C. make the experience expensive
    D. leave the basic problem unsolved

5. Of the following, the LEADING cause of *all* adult deaths is   5._____

    A. malignant neoplasms
    B. influenza and pneumonia
    C. heart disease
    D. vascular lesions of the central nervous system

6. Of the following, an overdose of insulin is MOST likely to produce   6._____

    A. nervousness, excessive hunger, weakness and sweating
    B. vomiting, labored respiration and anorexia
    C. polyuria, restlessness and anhydremia
    D. nausea, labored respiration and dyspnea

7. In essential hypertension, there is a(n)

   A. *increase* in systolic pressure and a *decrease* in diastolic pressure
   B. *decrease* in systolic pressure and an *increase* in diastolic pressure
   C. *increase* in *both* systolic and diastolic pressure
   D. *decrease* in *both* systolic and diastolic pressure

8. The use of mineral oil in low caloric diets should be discouraged CHIEFLY because it

   A. interferes with the absorption of all fat soluble vitamins
   B. spoils the flavor of food
   C. contains 9 calories per gram
   D. interferes with the absorption of sugar

9. Water is important in the daily intake of the body CHIEFLY because it

   A. causes the oxidation of food in the body
   B. is a transporting medium for all body substances
   C. cools the air in the lungs
   D. promotes protein metabolism

10. Of the following, the MOST important reason why a nurse should have a basic knowledge of the foods of the foreign-born is that

    A. many foreign dishes are more nutritious than American foods
    B. such knowledge would prove beyond doubt that poor diet is the cause of poor health among the foreign-born
    C. such knowledge would help the nurse to advise the patient on how to follow the prescribed diet using familiar foods
    D. it is interesting and exciting to eat the exotic dishes of foreign lands

11. Liver should be included in the diet chiefly because it is a GOOD source of

    A. Vitamin C   B. phosphorus   C. iodine   D. iron

12. Lack of iodine in the diet may result in

    A. gout   B. simple goiter
    C. arthritis   D. diabetes

13. The one of the following diseases which is the MOST COMMON cause of disability is

    A. arthritis   B. diabetes
    C. poliomyelitis   D. Parkinson's Disease

14. The glucose tolerance test is a test used to diagnose

    A. ulcers   B. hypertension
    C. leukemia   D. diabetes

15. When using a sphygmomanometer, the moment that the pulsation can be felt or heard marks the point of

    A. systolic blood pressure   B. diastolic blood pressure
    C. brachial stenosis   D. vasomotor restriction

16. The *initial* paralysis in cerebral vascular accident, regardless of cause, is the type known as

    A. spastic   B. paraplegic   C. flaccid   D. rigid

17. Cerebral hemorrhage *most frequently* occurs in males in the age range from

    A. 20 to 30 years
    B. 30 to 40 years
    C. 40 to 50 years
    D. 50 years and over

18. The one of the following conditions which is due to dysfunction of the thyroid gland is

    A. cholecystitis
    B. cretinism
    C. dwarfism
    D. epilepsy

19. The morbidity rate of tuberculosis is HIGHEST in the age range from

    A. birth to 20 years
    B. 20 to 45 years
    C. 45 to 65 years
    D. 65 years and over

20. An IMPORTANT early sign of carcinoma of the larynx is

    A. chronic hoarseness
    B. regurgitation of fluids
    C. difficulty in swallowing
    D. respiratory distress

21. Of the following, the MOST common and earliest recognizable sign of cancer of the breast is

    A. pain in the breast
    B. nipple discharge
    C. lump in the breast
    D. enlargement of the breast

22. In cancer of the breast, the lesion is MOST frequently found in the

    A. lower outer quadrant
    B. lower inner quadrant
    C. upper inner quadrant
    D. upper outer quadrant

23. Of the following, the MOST usual cause of hemoptysis in a 40-year-old male is

    A. tuberculosis
    B. cancer of the lung
    C. congenital ringworm
    D. spontaneous pneumothorax

24. Assume that a cardiac patient regularly assigned for nursing care has been receiving digitalis orally. On one of the nurse's regular home visits she finds the patient's radial pulse rate is 58. Nursing orders do not give specific directions regarding pulse.
    In this situation, it would be MOST advisable for the nurse to

    A. give no direction to the patient regarding medication but watch his pulse rate more closely on future visits for changes
    B. advise the patient to stop taking medication and tell him that she will report the pulse rate immediately to his physician
    C. report immediately to the physician on her observations as to pulse rate as well as regularity of pulse, patient's appetite, presence or absence of nausea
    D. teach the patient how to take his pulse and instruct hiiri to take digitalis if his pulse rate goes above 60

25. Hereditary progressive muscular dystrophy is a disease characterized by progressive weakness and final atrophy of groups of muscles.
Of the following statements about muscular dystrophy, the one which is LEAST accurate is that

   A. there is no known cure for muscular dystrophy at present
   B. muscular dystrophy is a disease of the central nervous system
   C. early signs of muscular dystrophy are frequent falls, difficulty climbing stairs, development of lordosis and a waddling gait
   D. therapeutic exercises may have some temporary value in the treatment of muscular dystrophy

26. The home care program is an extension of the hospital's service into the home on an extra-mural basis.
Of the following statements, the one that BEST explains the success of this program is that it

   A. recognizes the value to the patient and his family of the preservation of normal family life despite the limitations imposed by the patient's illness
   B. makes more hospital beds available for acute illnesses and emergency care
   C. reduces the cost of hospital care by reducing the number of in-patients
   D. simplifies hospital administration by reducing the number of chronically ill in hospitals

27. The PRIMARY objective of a day care program is to

   A. provide group care for a child in order to promote his physical or emotional adjustment
   B. insure adequate care, supervision and guidance for a child while his parents are at work
   C. safeguard a child's home and strengthen and support the family relationships for the child
   D. give financial assistance to voluntary agencies sponsoring the day care program

28. The MOST important of the following reasons for the rehabilitation of the seriously handicapped individual is that

   A. hospitalization of the handicapped is usually prolonged and costly to the community
   B. beds occupied by such patients reduce the number of hospital beds available for acutely ill patients
   C. care of chronically ill or handicapped patients is taxing and difficult for the family, the nurse and the doctor
   D. it is important to the patient that he be as independent and useful as possible

29. There has been a notable increase in the discharge rate from mental institutions in the state during recent years.
This change in statistics may be attributed CHIEFLY to

   A. increasing use of psychoanalysis and better trained personnel
   B. new drugs, changes in admission procedures and the "open door" policy
   C. the increase in nursing homes for the elderly
   D. the use of psychotherapeutics and early diagnosis of mental illness

30. The PRINCIPAL and BASIC objective of mental hygiene is to
    A. modify attitudes as well as unhealthy behavior secondary to unhealthy attitudes
    B. care for the post-hospitalized psychiatric patient at home
    C. increase mental hygiene clinic services
    D. stimulate interest in improved education for doctors, nurses and teachers

KEY (CORRECT ANSWERS)

1.	C	16.	C
2.	B	17.	D
3.	B	18.	B
4.	D	19.	D
5.	C	20.	A
6.	A	21.	C
7.	C	22.	D
8.	A	23.	A
9.	B	24.	C
10.	C	25.	B
11.	D	26.	A
12.	B	27.	C
13.	A	28.	D
14.	D	29.	B
15.	A	30.	A

TEST 2

DIRECTIONS: Each question or incomplete statement is followed by several suggested answers or completions. Select the one that BEST answers the question or completes the statement. *PRINT THE LETTER OF THE CORRECT ANSWER IN THE SPACE AT THE RIGHT.*

1. The incidence of syphilis is reported to be rising among teenagers in this country and the disease is still considered to be a major public health problem. Of the following statements about syphilis, the one which is NOT true is that   1.____

    A. the treatment most frequently used is penicillin
    B. at one stage of the disease, it causes a skin rash and enlarged lymph nodes
    C. the causative organism is the spirochete, treponema pallidum
    D. syphilis can be transmitted only by sexual intercourse

2. The one of the following which is the MOST dependable sign of pregnancy is   2.____

    A. fetal heart
    B. fetal movements felt by the mother
    C. a positive result on the Aschheim-Zondek test
    D. amenorrhea

3. An expectant mother states, "I did not plan this pregnancy and I am not making any preparations."   3.____
    Of the following, the BEST *initial* response for the nurse to make is:

    A. "Don't be upset. You will love your baby just the same."
    B. "Most mothers look forward to a lovely new baby."
    C. "Later when you feel differently you can make the necessary preparations."
    D. "It is not always easy to accept a pregnancy."

4. A nurse asks you to explain the significance of the Rh negative factor because she is concerned about one of her cases, an expectant mother who is Rh negative.   4.____
    Of the following, the BEST explanation you could give to this nurse is that

    A. Rh negative is a serious condition in the mother, frequently causing toxic symptoms
    B. if the father is Rh positive, there is no danger to either the mother or the baby
    C. if the baby should be positive, it may be adversely affected by the antibodies from the mother
    D. there is little danger with the Rh factor today because the mother can be treated to prevent the formation of antibodies

5. A mother who is 7-months pregnant tells the nurse that for the past few days she has been feeling dizzy and has had spots before her eyes. She has an appointment to see her doctor in a week.   5.____
    Of the following, the BEST advice for the nurse to give this mother is to

    A. not be alarmed but report this to the doctor at her next appointment
    B. rest at least two hours each day and avoid exertion
    C. limit the amount of fluid intake to 3-4 glasses daily
    D. either call the doctor or go to the hospital immediately

6. Assume that a newly appointed nurse asks you what she should do if she were to find, on one of her regular visits, that a mother was in advanced labor.
   Of the following, the BEST advice for you to give the nurse is that, in this situation, she should

   A. go out to the nearest telephone booth and call for an ambulance
   B. apply gentle pressure to the uterus
   C. encourage the mother to bear down
   D. support the baby's head and body as they are delivered

7. To meet the calcium requirement during the second half of pregnancy, it is recommended that the diet of a pregnant woman contain

   A. at least two eggs daily
   B. one quart of milk daily
   C. a serving of liver twice weekly
   D. at least two oranges daily

8. A mother seven months pregnant with her first baby asks the nurse how she will know when to go to the hospital.
   Of the following, the BEST response is that she should go to the hospital when

   A. the membranes rupture, whether or not she has contractions
   B. she has a mucus vaginal discharge
   C. the baby shows marked increase in activity
   D. the baby sinks down into the pelvis and she feels pressure on the bladder and rectum

9. During an in-service education session, a nurse asks for additional information about pre-eclamptic toxemia.
   Of the following, the MOST accurate information you could give this nurse is that

   A. toxemia usually occurs during the first trimester of pregnancy
   B. overexertion on the part of the mother is known to cause toxemia
   C. pre-eclamptic toxemia is a preventable condition whose cause is well known and well understood
   D. this condition is usually marked by headache, nausea and vomiting

10. A young nurse asks you how she can help a mother who is breast feeding her baby but does not have a sufficient amount of milk.
    Of the following, the *most helpful* suggestion the nurse could make to this mother is:

    A. "Nurse the baby every other feeding. This will allow the breasts to fill up between feedings."
    B. "Plenty of rest and good food will insure a good supply of milk."
    C. "Have the baby empty the breasts completely and regularly before supplementing with the bottle."
    D. "Many women are too nervous to successfully breast feed."

11. A mother who is 3 months *post partum* has been nursing her baby. She tells the nurse that she has not menstruated and asks if it is possible that she is now pregnant.
    Of the following, the BEST answer the nurse could give to this mother is:

A. "You cannot become pregnant while you nurse your baby."
B. "You cannot be pregnant until you have your first menstrual period."
C. "You may become pregnant at any time if you have intercourse."
D. "You cannot become pregnant until your uterus has completely involuted."

12. The OUTSTANDING cause of death during the first twenty-four hours of life is

    A. congenital anomalies B. prematurity
    C. atelectasis D. erythroblastosis

13. Of the following, the one which is LEAST characteristic of the eyes of a normal newborn child is that

    A. the pupils contract in bright light
    B. sight is confined to the ability to distinguish light from darkness
    C. the lachrymal glands secrete fluid
    D. bright light causes closure of the eyelids

14. Of the following reflexes, the one which is NOT normal in a month-old infant is

    A. drawing up the legs when startled
    B. grasping an article placed in its hand
    C. sucking
    D. ability to focus the eyes

15. Of the following signs, the one which is MOST helpful in the early diagnosis of congenital hip dislocation in the newborn is

    A. marked hip prominence
    B. an even number of gluteal folds
    C. an uneven number of gluteal folds
    D. a grating sound on movement of the hips

16. Egg yolk from a hard cooked egg is added to an infant's diet at the age of three months CHIEFLY to

    A. compensate for the low iron content of milk
    B. give bulk to the diet
    C. add protein to the diet
    D. compensate for the low fat content of milk

17. Kicking in a six-month-old baby is *usually* a(n)

    A. expression of bad temper
    B. sign of excessive restlessness
    C. normal muscular activity which may be a preparation for walking
    D. attempt to attract the attention of the nearest adult

18. Of the following statements with respect to the nutritional needs of children, the one which is MOST accurate is that

    A. a four-year-old child requires a minimum of 2000 calories a day
    B. proportionately, children require more protein per pound of body weight than do adults

C. it is better for a child to be slightly underweight than to be overweight
D. a child whose diet is deficient in Vitamin D may develop scurvy as a result

19. Cod liver oil is given to children CHIEFLY in order to aid in

    A. absorption of calcium
    B. carbohydrate metabolism
    C. prevention of beriberi
    D. regulation of osmotic pressure

20. The LEADING cause of death in this country for children from one to four years of age is

    A. influenza and pneumonia
    B. congenital malformations
    C. malignant neoplasms of blood and lymph
    D. accidents

21. Reconstructive surgery for cleft palate SHOULD be done

    A. at about one month of age
    B. before the child begins to talk
    C. when the child is six months old
    D. when explanation of the procedure can be understood by the child

22. Separation of a child from his own home and placement in a foster home often arouses adverse reactions in the child.
    Of the following, the one which is MOST serious for the child is

    A. homesickness
    B. withdrawn behavior
    C. rebellion against authority
    D. dislike of new people

23. Behavior problems of the adolescent school child can BEST be explained by the fact that

    A. the adolescent suddenly becomes aware of the opposite sex at this time
    B. the demands made on adolescents by intolerant parents create rebellion against authority
    C. during childhood there is a general disregard of the child's need for independence by parents and other adults
    D. adolescence is a transition period between childhood and adulthood which usually creates feelings of insecurity in the adolescent

24. Of the following, the behavior which is LEAST indicative of serious emotional maladjustment in an adolescent boy is

    A. lying and cheating
    B. shyness and daydreaming
    C. gross overweight
    D. association with a teenage gang

25. The precipitating cause of dental caries is

    A. inadequate cleaning of teeth by toothbrushing
    B. failure to maintain a daily diet containing all of the essential food elements in the right amounts
    C. decalcification of the tooth enamel by acids produced in the fermentation of carbohydrates
    D. inherited differences in the ability to resist caries

26. For GREATEST effectiveness, topical application of a fluorine solution should be started

    A. as soon as possible after the deciduous teeth erupt
    B. when the child enters the first grade in school
    C. on the child's first visit to the dentist
    D. when the permanent teeth have erupted

27. The MOST important one of the following contributions that the school nurse can make to the effort to conserve sight and to prevent eye strain in the classroom is to

    A. advise the principal to have the walls painted a light color so as to diffuse the light throughout the classroom
    B. determine whether the school office has in its files the accepted standards for classroom lighting
    C. instruct the teacher and students regarding proper seating and utilization of light in the classroom
    D. provide the teacher with a list of all students in her class who test 20/40 or more on the visual acuity test

28. Of the following statements concerning eyeglasses, the one which is LEAST accurate is that glasses are prescribed in order to

    A. cure infectious diseases of the eye
    B. improve vision and relieve eyestrain
    C. neutralize defects of focus of the eyes
    D. strengthen weak eye muscles

29. Of the following, the BEST description of early symptoms of glaucoma is dimness in visual acuity,

    A. and marked itching of the eyelids
    B. with or without pain in the eye
    C. and haloed lights, with or without pain in the eye
    D. marked itching and redness of the sclera and eyelids

30. Unequal arm or leg lengths, or differences in shoulder height with scapular protrusion, are *early* manifestations of

    A. kyphosis   B. scoliosis   C. torticollis   D. lordosis

KEY (CORRECT ANSWERS)

1. D
2. A
3. D
4. C
5. D

6. D
7. B
8. A
9. D
10. C

11. C
12. B
13. C
14. D
15. C

16. A
17. C
18. B
19. A
20. D

21. B
22. B
23. D
24. D
25. C

26. A
27. C
28. A
29. C
30. B

EXAMINATION SECTION
TEST 1

DIRECTIONS: Each question or incomplete statement is followed by several suggested answers or completions. Select the one that *BEST* answers the question or completes the statement. *PRINT THE LETTER OF THE CORRECT ANSWER IN THE SPACE AT THE RIGHT.*

1. Neonatal respiratory distress in which the alveoli and the alveolar ducts are filled with a sticky exudate preventing aeration is known as   1.____

    A. caput succedaneum
    B. atelectasis
    C. cephalhematoma
    D. hyaline membrane disease

2. Concerning nutrition, the *PRIMARY* role of the nurse is to   2.____

    A. change the food patterns of the home
    B. help a patient follow the doctor's orders
    C. teach basic principles of food selection
    D. assist in food selection for the family

3. In an aortogram study of extracranial vessels, introduction of the catheter into the femoral artery is *preferable* because it visualizes   3.____

    A. external carotids and branches
    B. temporal artery and branches
    C. femoral artery and branches
    D. aortic artery and branches

4. The *CHIEF* substance used in aortography are compounds of   4.____

    A. Iodine
    B. Sulfa
    C. Silver
    D. Carbon

5. The technique for artificial respiration that has the advantage of providing pressure to inflate the victim's lungs *immediately* is the _____ method.   5.____

    A. back-pressure arm-lift
    B. chest-pressure arm-lift
    C. mouth-to-mouth
    D. prone-posture

6. Repeated attacks of hypoglycemia in diabetic children receiving insulin may produce   6.____

    A. acidosis
    B. brain damage
    C. diabetic coma
    D. ketosis

7. An antiviral protein produced by cells infected with virus which may prove to be an *effective* therapy in virus infections is   7.____

    A. beta globulin
    B. RNA
    C. gamma globulin
    D. interferon

8. The *DIRECT* source of muscle energy is   8.____

    A. potassium phosphate
    B. lactic acid
    C. sarcolactic acid
    D. phosphocreatin

9. The vitamin *essential* for the synthesis of prothrombin is

   A. P B. B1 C. B6 D. K

10. Tubes containing radium are disinfected when necessary by

    A. boiling to 212°
    B. boiling to 250°
    C. heat under pressure
    D. chemical disinfection

11. The cardinal symptoms of erythroblastosis are:

    A. Cherry red nail beds and coughing
    B. Paroxysms of coughing and labored breathing
    C. Jaundice and anemia
    D. Dehydration and marked thirst

12. A hypertensive patient with cardiovascular-renal complications *usually* is advised to eat a _____ diet.

    A. Meulengracht B. Brecht C. high sodium D. low sodium

13. Wilm's Tumor, often found in children, is a disease of the

    A. brain B. kidney C. duodenum D. liver

14. In the phenylketonuric child, the diet must be limited in

    A. phenolphthalein B. phenylalanine
    C. phenylhydrazine D. phenylkania

15. A patient with a hemorrhage from a peptic ulcer is sometimes placed on a(n) _____ diet.

    A. Andresen B. gluten-free
    C. low gelatin glucose D. nutramigen

16. A *distinguishing* feature of the Jacksonian form of epilepsy is the

    A. convulsive muscular behavior
    B. involvement of only one side of the body
    C. momentary lapse of consciousness
    D. presence of psychic disturbances

17. Bacteriological sanitary analysis is made PRIMARILY to determine the presence of

    A. colon bacillus B. disease germs
    C. nitrates D. spore-forming bacteria

18. The *BEST* sources of the vitamin that is important to coagulation are:

    A. Beef liver, calf liver, chicken liver
    B. Cabbage, cauliflower, spinach
    C. Corn, peas, yellow beans
    D. Grapes, melon, pears

19. The *key* constituent of the thyroid hormone is   19.____

    A. fluorine   B. iodine   C. chlorine   D. thyrine

20. The *daily* requirement of thiamine for an adult is   20.____

    A. related to the amount of carbohydrate being metabolized
    B. 8.4 mg.
    C. .006 mg.
    D. related to the amount of fats being hydrolyzed

21. In liver diseases, such as infectious hepatitis, the diet must be modified to   21.____

    A. *increase* roughage   B. *decrease* carbohydrates
    C. *increase* fat content   D. *increase* protein intake

22. Distilled water added to a drop of blood on a slide will cause the erythrocytes to   22.____

    A. agglutinate   B. crenate
    C. shrivel   D. swell

23. Following early diagnosis of galactosemia, the health of the child is protected by keeping the diet *free* of   23.____

    A. eggs   B. meat   C. milk   D. potatoes

24. Friedman's Test is a   24.____

    A. modification of the A-Z test
    B. blood sugar tolerance test
    C. renal function test
    D. Vitamin K test

25. Aldosterone, the hormone essential for normal retention of sodium and excretion of potassium, is secreted by the   25.____

    A. adrenal cortex   B. parathyroids
    C. gonads   D. pituitary

KEY (CORRECT ANSWERS)

1. D
2. B
3. D
4. A
5. C

6. B
7. D
8. D
9. D
10. D

11. C
12. D
13. B
14. B
15. A

16. B
17. A
18. B
19. B
20. A

21. D
22. D
23. C
24. A
25. A

TEST 2

DIRECTIONS: Each question or incomplete statement is followed by several suggested answers or completions. Select the one that BEST answers the question or completes the statement. PRINT THE LETTER OF THE CORRECT ANSWER IN THE SPACE AT THE RIGHT.

1. The coat of viruses consists of

   A. enzymes
   B. nucleic acids
   C. polysaccharides
   D. protein

   1._____

2. Of the following, the *one* that is NOT a symptom of radiation sickness is

   A. bleeding from mucous membranes
   B. breathing difficulty
   C. diarrhea
   D. sore throat

   2._____

3. The rate of oxidation of alcohol in the body is

   A. accelerated by exercise
   B. fixed
   C. retarded by exercise
   D. retarded by sleep

   3._____

4. A "broad-spectrum" antibiotic is

   A. bacitracin
   B. streptomycin
   C. chrysomycin
   D. aureomycin

   4._____

5. If a virus were seen outside the living cell, it would appear to be

   A. non-living
   B. parasitic
   C. saprophytic
   D. toxic

   5._____

6. Slight exposure to radioactive dust will cause

   A. destruction of germ cells
   B. destruction of brain tissue
   C. severe illness
   D. skin burns

   6._____

7. A xanthine diuretic is

   A. caffeine
   B. calomel
   C. acetazolamide
   D. trichlormethiazide

   7._____

8. An organism that grows rapidly in many foods and is the MOST common cause of gastro-intestinal infection is

   A. clostridium botulism
   B. dysentery bacillus
   C. salmonella
   D. streptococcus

   8._____

9. Indiscriminate use of Vitamin D may lead to

   A. hearing loss
   B. excess bone calcification
   C. calcification of the arteries of the heart
   D. increase of the anti-menorrhagic factor in blood

   9._____

33

10. In nutrition, increasing attention is being given to the importance of

   A. carbohydrates B. vitamins
   C. minerals D. amino acids

11. Sufferers from silcosis have turned increasingly to

   A. streptomycin B. chlorine gas
   C. silicic acid D. powdered aluminum

12. The medical term used to describe simple goiter is

   A. simple adenoma B. myxedema
   C. colloid goiter D. hyperthyroidism

13. What is considered to be the normal polymorphonuclear count?

   A. 80 - 100%   B. 70 - 80%   C. 60 - 70%   D. 50 - 60%

14. The range of normal metabolism is *generally* considered to be:

   A. minus 5 to plus 5 B. minus 10 to plus 10
   C. minus 20, to plus 20 D. minus 25 to plus 25

15. If a patient ate everything served him for breakfast except 10 grams of bacon, his caloric intake for this meal would be decreased by _____ calories.

   A. 10   B. 40   C. 60   D. 90

16. If you were asked to prepare one quart of 1-1000 solution of mercuric chloride from tablets 0.5 grams, *how many* tablets would you use?

   A. 2   B. 5   C. 7 1/2   D. 13

17. The discomfort of constipation is due to

   A. pressure of the fecal material on the rectum
   B. absorption of toxins from the colon
   C. increased bacterial content in the colon
   D. gases produced by the bacillus coli

18. The *one BEST* explanation why soap and water are more effective in cleansing than clear water is that

   A. soap softens the water
   B. clear water adheres more closely to the surface of an object
   C. the surface tension of a soap-and-water solution is lower than that of clear water
   D. clear water promotes absorption

19. In the care of a patient with communicable disease in the home, the *accepted* method for the care of his dishes is:

   A. Wash in the sink
   B. Wash in the sink and boil
   C. Boil and then wash in the sink
   D. Soak in a disinfectant solution and then wash

20. Of the following superficial body areas, the one that would be affected *early* by a diet deficient in niacin is the

    A. cornea   B. conjunctiva   C. gums   D. tongue

21. The *MOST* effective method for cleaning contaminated hands is washing with soap

    A. and hot running water
    B. and water in a basin
    C. hot running water, and a sterile brush
    D. in hot running water, and rinsing in a 70%-solution of alcohol

22. In a *second-degree* burn, the *DEEPEST* tissue affected is the

    A. epidermis   B. dermis
    C. subcutaneous tissue   D. muscle

23. The *MOST* desirable first-aid treatment for burns is the use of

    A. tannic acid jelly   B. tannic acid spray
    C. vaseline   D. sodium bicarbonate paste

24. An *inexpensive* food source of iron is

    A. potato   B. carrots   C. milk   D. meat

25. One of the substances which is added to "enriched" bread is

    A. Vitamin A   B. thiamin   C. ascorbic acid   D. niacin

KEY (CORRECT ANSWERS)

1. D		11. D	
2. B		12. C	
3. B		13. C	
4. D		14. B	
5. A		15. B	
6. D		16. A	
7. A		17. A	
8. C		18. C	
9. B		19. D	
10. D		20. D	

21. D
22. B
23. C
24. A
25. B

EXAMINATION SECTION
TEST 1

DIRECTIONS: Each question or incomplete statement is followed by several suggested answers or completions. Select the one that BEST answers the question or completes the statement. *PRINT THE LETTER OF THE CORRECT ANSWER IN THE SPACE AT THE RIGHT.*

1. An employee should know not only the details of his own job but the main objective of the organization for which he works.
   The MAIN objective of a health center may BEST be described as the

   A. orderly and efficient management of the health center
   B. improvement of the health of the community it serves
   C. courteous treatment of patients who are poor
   D. enforcement of the health laws of the city

2. The MOST appropriate of the following statements for Miss Smith, who works in the cardiac clinic, to make when answering the clinic telephone is:

   A. This is the Cardiac Clinic. Who's calling please?
   B. Hello. This is Miss Smith.
   C. Cardiac Clinic, Miss Smith speaking. May I help you?
   D. Miss Smith speaking. To whom do you wish to speak?

3. Of the following, the CHIEF reason why you should be familiar with medical terminology is so that you can

   A. be of greatest assistance to the doctors and nurses
   B. answer the patient's questions about their symptoms and treatments
   C. know what supplies to order for the clinic
   D. understand the medical publications which are sent to the clinic

4. Assume that instructions have been issued in your clinic that medical information is not to be given to patients. Of the following, the BEST reason for this policy is that

   A. the relationship between the clinic staff and clinic patients, although friendly, should remain impersonal
   B. the health of a patient is a private matter which should not be discussed in public
   C. incorrect medical information might be given to the patient
   D. only the nurse in charge should be permitted to give medical information to patients

5. Of the following, the BEST reason for keeping clinic records confidential is to

   A. protect the patient who may not want others to know certain information
   B. protect the health station in case errors have been made
   C. prevent publicity about the health station which may keep patients from coming to the clinics
   D. avoid the extra work involved in giving out information

6. To give each patient who is to return to the clinic a card with the date of his next appointment written on it is

A. unnecessary; it is sufficient to tell him when to come back
B. of little value; some of the patients may not be able to read English
C. impractical; too much time would be taken up in writing the cards
D. good practice; the patient would be less likely to forget his next date

7. When setting up a *tickler* file for patients' appointments in your clinic, you should arrange the cards according to the

   A. name of the patient
   B. date when the patient is due in the clinic
   C. condition for which the patient is being treated
   D. name of the doctor

8. Assume that you are responsible for maintaining the patients' record file in the clinic to which you are assigned. Frequently, the other clinics in the health center where you work borrow record cards from your clinic files.
   The BEST way for you to avoid difficulty in locating cards which may have been borrowed by other clinics is to

   A. make out a duplicate card for any clinic that wishes to borrow a card from your file
   B. refuse to lend your card to any other clinic unless the other clinic's personnel officer promises to return the card in person
   C. report it to your supervisor if anyone fails to return a card after a reasonable time
   D. have the person who borrows a card fill out an out-of-file card and place it in the file whenever a record card is removed

9. Suppose that you are given an unalphabetized list of 500 clinic patients and a set of unalphabetized record cards. Your supervisor asks you to determine if there is a record card for each patient whose name is on the list.
   For you to first arrange the record cards in alphabetical order before checking them with the names on the list is

   A. *desirable;* this will make it easier to check each name on the list against the patients' record cards
   B. *undesirable;* it is just as easy to alphabetize the names on the list as it is to rearrange the record cards
   C. *desirable;* this extra work with the record cards will give you more information about the patients
   D. *undesirable;* adding an extra step to the procedure makes the work too complicated

10. Suppose that you have been given about two thousand 3x5 cards to arrange in numerical order.
    For you to sort the cards into broad groups, such as 1-100, 101-200, etc., and then arrange each group of cards in numerical order is

    A. *desirable;* you will not be so apt to lose your place if interrupted when working with small groups of cards
    B. *undesirable;* setting up a large number of groups of cards leads to more errors
    C. *desirable;* the work can be done more quickly and easily with smaller groups of cards than with the entire group at once
    D. *undesirable;* any procedure which requires so many steps wastes too much time

11. Of the following, the MOST important reason for keeping accurate records of clinic patients is that

    A. these records provide valuable information for medical research purposes
    B. accurate records are necessary to provide satisfactory medical care for the patients on return visits
    C. complete records are necessary in order to prepare accurate and complete statistical reports on the work of the clinic
    D. these records will show the large amount of work performed in the clinic

12. Suppose that one of the doctors who has been seeing patients on Wednesday changes his clinic day to Thursday. Two women who have previously had Wednesday appointments ask to come in on Thursday because they have great confidence in this doctor. For you to try to make Thursday appointments for them would be

    A. *correct;* the wishes of the patients should be considered in making appointments
    B. *wrong;* if the request were granted, the other patients would also want to have their appointments changed
    C. *correct;* most patients would rather come to the clinic on Wednesdays
    D. *wrong;* patients should not become too dependent upon any one physician

13. Of the following, the CHIEF reason for paying attention to a complaint from a clinic patient is that

    A. government employees should always be courteous to the public
    B. most people like to have others pay attention to their complaints
    C. it does no harm to listen to complaints even if there is no merit to them
    D. the patient may have good reason to complain

14. Assume that it is the rule in the clinic that the doctor is to sign the personal record card of each patient he examines. While you are filing the patients' record cards after the doctor has left the clinic, you notice that he has not signed the card of one of the patients he examined. Of the following, the MOST appropriate action for you to take is to

    A. sign your own name on the card since the doctor has left the clinic
    B. write the doctor's name on the card and sign your initials
    C. file the unsigned card in the record file with the other cards
    D. hold the card out and return it to the doctor for his signature on his next visit

15. Assume that it is the rule in the clinic that no patient may be seen after 4:00 P.M. so that the physicians and nurses will have time to write up cases and prepare for the following day. A few minutes after 4:00 P.M., an old woman who says she is in great pain and discomfort appears and asks for a doctor.
    For you to try to arrange for a physician to see her is

    A. *proper;* other patients waiting in the clinic will see how kind you are to sick people
    B. *improper;* a rule should never be broken by public health personnel
    C. *proper;* rules should not be interpreted too strictly when dealing with sick people
    D. *improper;* the physician would be very annoyed if you disturbed him after 4:00 P.M.

16. Assume that you have been instructed to note on the record of each child who is vaccinated the lot number of the vaccine used.
    Of the following, the MOST probable reason for this instruction is so that

A. a record can be kept of how much vaccine is used every year
B. if the child has an unfavorable reaction, the lot may be tested to determine the reason
C. no child will receive more than one vaccination
D. the oldest vaccine will be used first

17. The mother of a young child who is to be vaccinated against smallpox informs you that he gets hysterical at the sight of a needle.
Of the following, the BEST thing for you to do is to

   A. assure the mother that the child's fears are groundless
   B. speak to the child about the need to be protected against a serious disease like smallpox
   C. tell the head nurse about the child's fear before he is called for vaccination
   D. promise the child a lollypop or toy if he behaves and does not cry

18. A 10-year-old boy who is grossly overweight refuses to remove any of his clothing before being weighed, apparently because of embarrassment.
Of the following, it is BEST for you to

   A. weigh him fully dressed and note this fact on the record
   B. insist that he remove his clothing since otherwise the record would be inaccurate
   C. note on the record card *grossly overweight,* as you cannot weigh him with his clothing
   D. ask the head nurse to use her authority to make the boy undress

19. You notice that an 8-year-old boy who attends the clinic stammers badly.
Of the following, it is BEST for you to

   A. tell the doctor about his stammering in the boy's presence
   B. tell the boy each time you see him that his speech has improved
   C. ask the boy if he would like to go to a speech correction clinic
   D. make no reference to his stammer in the boy's presence

20. Of the following, the MOST important reason why you should remain with a 4-year-old child when his temperature is being taken by mouth is that otherwise the child might

   A. fall off the chair and fracture an arm or leg
   B. break the thermometer while it is in his mouth
   C. remove the thermometer from his mouth and misplace it
   D. leave the examining room and return to his mother

21. The BEST way to take the temperature of an infant is by

   A. feeling his forehead
   B. using an oral thermometer
   C. placing a thermometer under his armpit
   D. using a rectal thermometer

22. When the temperature of an adult is taken rectally, it is LEAST accurate to say that the

   A. temperature reading will be higher than if it were taken orally
   B. thermometer should be lubricated before use

C. thermometer should be in place for at least ten minutes
D. temperature reading is likely to be more accurate than if it were taken orally

23. When the temperature of an adult is taken orally, it is LEAST accurate to say that the

    A. thermometer should be washed with alcohol before it is used
    B. thermometer should be taken down below 96° F before it is used
    C. patient's temperature may be taken immediately after he has smoked a cigarette
    D. patient should be inactive just before his temperature is taken

24. The nurse described the test to the patient before bringing him to the examining room for a basal metabolism test.
    Her action may BEST be described as

    A. *correat;* the patient will be more cooperative if he knows what to expect
    B. *wrong;* the nurse does not know how the test will affect the patient
    C. *correct;* the nurse can judge whether the patient is too upset by this information to take the test
    D. *wrong;* explaining the test beforehand will only make the patient nervous

25. When a patient's sputum test is *positive*, it means that the

    A. patient's sputum is plentiful
    B. doctor has made an accurate diagnosis
    C. patient has recovered and is now in good health
    D. laboratory reports that the patient's sputum contains certain disease germs

26. A biopsy can BEST be described as a(n)

    A. pre-cancerous condition   B. examination of tissues
    C. living organism   D. germicidal solution

27. The *scratch* or *patch* test is usually given when testing for

    A. allergies   B. rheumatic fever
    C. blood poisoning   D. diabetes

28. Gamma globulin is frequently given to children after exposure to and before the appearance of symptoms of

    A. measles   B. smallpox
    C. tetanus   D. chickenpox

29. Of the following, the one which is NOT a respiratory disease is

    A. bronchitis   B. pneumonia
    C. nephritis   D. croup

30. A physician who specializes in the treatment of conditions affecting the skin is known as a

    A. urologist   B. dermatologist
    C. toxicologist   D. ophthalmologist

31. The branch of medicine which deals with diseases peculiar to women is

   A. pathology
   B. orthopedics
   C. neurology
   D. gynecology

32. The branch of medicine which deals with diseases of old age is called

   A. pediatrics
   B. geriatrics
   C. serology
   D. histology

33. *Petit mal* is a form of

   A. epilepsy
   B. syphilis
   C. diabetes
   D. malaria

34. Glaucoma is a disease of the

   A. thyroid gland
   B. liver
   C. bladder
   D. eye

35. A patient who has edema has

   A. not enough red blood cells
   B. too much water in the body tissues
   C. blood in the urine
   D. a swollen gland

36. The thoracic area of the body is located in the

   A. abdomen
   B. lower back
   C. chest
   D. neck

37. An electrocardiograph is MOST usually used in examination of the

   A. brain
   B. heart
   C. kidney
   D. gall bladder

38. The word *coagulate* means MOST NEARLY to

   A. bleed excessively
   B. break up
   C. work together
   D. form a clot

39. A stethoscope is used to examine the patient's

   A. heart
   B. patellar reflex
   C. blood cells
   D. spinal fluid

40. A pelvimeter is MOST usually used in the examination of a patient in the _____ clinic.

   A. chest   B. cancer   C. prenatal   D. eye

41. Tuberculin may BEST be described as a

   A. virus infection of the lungs
   B. preparation used in the diagnosis of tuberculosis
   C. sanitarium for tuberculous patients
   D. form of cancer of the lung

42. An autoclave is a(n)

    A. automatic dispenser of instruments needed for clinic examinations
    B. sterile place for storing clinic supplies until they are needed
    C. apparatus for sterilizing equipment under steam pressure
    D. portable self-operating general anesthesia unit

43. Radiation therapy is

    A. the recording of electrical impulses of the body on a graph
    B. a study of the effects of radiation fall-out on the human body
    C. a form of treatment used for certain diseases
    D. the filming of internal parts of the body through the use of x-rays

44. Diathermy is the treatment of patients by

    A. scientific use of baths and mineral waters
    B. insertion of radium into diseased tissues
    C. intravenous feedings of vitamins and minerals
    D. electrical generation of heat in the body tissues

45. The measurement of blood pressure involves two readings, which are known as _____ and _____.

    A. metabolic; diastolic
    B. systolic; diastolic
    C. metabolic; hyperbolic
    D. hyperbolic; systolic

46. The Snellen chart is used in examinations of the

    A. eyes
    B. blood
    C. urine
    D. bile

47. An enema is MOST generally used to

    A. induce vomiting
    B. irrigate the stomach
    C. clear the bowels
    D. drain the urinary bladder

48. A bronchoscope is usually used in examinations of the

    A. kidneys
    B. heart
    C. stomach
    D. lungs

49. The Wassermann test is used to find out if a patient has

    A. diphtheria
    B. leukemia
    C. scarlet fever
    D. syphilis

50. If a boiling water sterilizer is used, the minimum time necessary to sterilize instruments is MOST NEARLY _____ hour(s).

    A. 1/2
    B. 1
    C. 1 1/2
    D. 2

KEY (CORRECT ANSWERS)

1. B	11. B	21. D	31. D	41. B
2. C	12. A	22. C	32. B	42. C
3. A	13. D	23. C	33. A	43. C
4. C	14. D	24. A	34. D	44. D
5. A	15. C	25. D	35. B	45. B
6. D	16. B	26. B	36. C	46. A
7. B	17. C	27. A	37. B	47. C
8. D	18. A	28. A	38. D	48. D
9. A	19. D	29. C	39. A	49. D
10. C	20. B	30. B	40. C	50. A

TEST 2

DIRECTIONS: Each question or incomplete statement is followed by several suggested answers or completions. Select the one that BEST answers the question or completes the statement. *PRINT THE LETTER OF THE CORRECT ANSWER IN THE SPACE AT THE RIGHT.*

1. To sterilize towels and dry gauze dressings in the health clinic, it is MOST advisable to   1.____

    A. dip them in a sterilizing solution
    B. wash them with a strong detergent
    C. boil them in the sterilizer
    D. steam them under pressure

2. Sterilization by use of chemicals rather than by boiling water is indicated when the instrument   2.____

    A. is made of soft rubber
    B. has a sharp cutting edge
    C. has pus or blood on it
    D. was used more than 24 hours before sterilization

3. When dusting the furniture in the clinic, it is advisable to use a silicone-treated dustcloth CHIEFLY because the treated cloth will   3.____

    A. collect the dust more efficiently
    B. disinfect as well as dust the furniture
    C. not remove the wax from the furniture
    D. make it unnecessary to polish the furniture in the future

4. Assume that the clinic in which you work has issued instructions that all supplies containing poison are to have blue labels with the word *poison* clearly marked on the label, and that these supplies are to be kept in a storage cabinet separate from other supplies. You notice that a bottle with no label is on a shelf in the *poison* storage cabinet.
Of the following, the BEST action for you to take is to   4.____

    A. place the unlabeled bottle in the back of the regular storage cabinet
    B. put a blue label on the bottle and write *poison* on the label
    C. ask another public health employee to help you decide if the bottle contains poison
    D. pour the contents of the bottle into the slop sink and destroy the bottle

5. Assume that you have been assigned to care for the supply room, and have been instructed to use the items which have been in stock longest before using the newer stock. Of the following, the MOST practical and time-saving way to do this is to   5.____

    A. keep a record file of all supplies received and used
    B. write the dates when the supplies were received and used on the labels or containers
    C. place new supplies behind supplies of the same items already in stock
    D. keep the fastest moving stock in the most convenient places

6. The public health employee should know that clinic supplies should be reordered
    A. as soon as the last container of the item in the supply closet is used up
    B. in the same amount on the first working day of each month
    C. whenever a let-up in clinic work makes time available
    D. when the records show that the stock may possibly be depleted within a month

7. The CHIEF reason for storing x-ray film in lead containers is that lead containers protect the film from
    A. moisture in the atmosphere
    B. exposure to stray x-rays
    C. dust and other particles
    D. extreme changes in temperature

8. You have been instructed to keep all narcotics locked in a separate cabinet when storing supplies.
   The one of the following which should be kept locked in this cabinet is a preparation containing
    A. cortisone   B. codeine   C. caffeine   D. quinine

9. Of the following medical supplies, the one which should be refrigerated is
    A. vaseline jelly   B. paregoric
    C. aureomycin   D. aspirin tablets

10. The one of the following which is NOT an antiseptic or disinfectant is
    A. distilled water   B. alcohol
    C. lysol   D. hydrogen peroxide

11. The one of the following which is an anesthetic is
    A. novocaine   B. phenobarbital
    C. benzedrine   D. witch hazel

12. The wide use of antibiotics has presented a number of problems. Some patients become allergic to the drugs so that they cannot be used when they are needed. In other cases, after prolonged treatment with antibiotics, certain organisms no longer respond to them at all. This is one of the reasons for the constant search for more potent drugs.
    On the basis of this paragraph, the one of the following statements which is MOST NEARLY correct is that
    A. antibiotics have been used successfully for certain allergies
    B. antibiotics should never be used for prolonged treatment
    C. because they have developed an allergy to the drug, antibiotics cannot be used when needed for certain patients
    D. one of the reasons for the constant search for new antibiotics is that so many diseases have been successfully treated with these drugs

13. The over-use of antibiotics today represents a growing danger, according to many medical authorities. Patients everywhere, stimulated by reports of new wonder drugs, continue to ask their doctors for a shot to relieve a cold, grippe, or any of the other virus infections that occur during the course of a bad winter. But, for the common cold and many other virus infections, antibiotics have no effect.
On the basis of this paragraph, the one of the following statements which is MOST NEARLY correct is that

    A. the use of antibiotics is becoming a health hazard
    B. antibiotics are of no value in the treatment of many virus infections
    C. patients should ask their doctors for a shot of one of the new wonder drugs to relieve the symptoms of grippe
    D. the treatment of colds and other virus infections by antibiotics will lessen their severity

14. Statistics tell us that heart disease kills more people than any other illness, and the death rate still continues to rise. People over 30 have a fifty-fifty chance of escaping, for heart disease is chiefly an illness of people in late middle age and advanced years. Because there are more people in this age group living today than there were some years ago, heart disease is able to find more victims.
On the basis of this paragraph, the one of the following statements which is MOST NEARLY correct is that

    A. half of the people over 30 years of age have heart disease today
    B. more people die of heart disease than of all other diseases combined
    C. older people are the chief victims of heart disease
    D. the rising birth rate has increased the possibility that the average person will die of heart disease

15. There is evidence that some individuals, given three doses of polio vaccine, have not developed enough immunity to protect themselves against paralytic polio. It is thought that immunity will be increased by a fourth injection given no sooner than one year after the third injection and many health agencies have been giving a fourth injection to their patients.
On the basis of this paragraph, the one of the following statements which is MOST NEARLY correct is that

    A. three doses of polio vaccine will not give any protection from paralytic polio
    B. a fourth injection of polio vaccine guarantees immunity to polio
    C. the fourth injection of polio vaccine should be given as soon as possible after the third injection
    D. the fourth injection of polio vaccine should be given at least a year after the third injection

Questions 16-22.

DIRECTIONS: Questions 16 through 22 are to be answered on the basis of the following table.

REPORT ON PATIENTS ATTENDING SELECTED HEALTH CLINICS January to December (This Year)					
CLINICS	A	B	C	D	E
Child Health	62,400	70,200	81,900	83,400	22,300
Chest	53,300	52,000	64,800	47,600	4,500
Social Hygiene	24,500	21,900	18,400	13,500	4,100
Eye	10,600	12,600	13,300	13,800	4,200
Cardiac	1,400	1,600	1,700	1,300	400
Prenatal	1,300	1,800	1,700	1,800	500

16. On the basis of the above chart, the group with the LARGEST number of patients attending the eye clinics was

    A. B B. C C. A D. D

17. If the population of the area located around group E was 210,000, the percentage of this population who attended the eye clinic was MOST NEARLY

    A. .02% B. 2% C. 5% D. 21%

18. If the clinics were open 250 days, the average daily attendance at the social hygiene clinics in group C was MOST NEARLY

    A. 74 B. 88 C. 259 D. 736

19. The percentage of all patients attending group E clinics who attended the chest clinics was MOST NEARLY

    A. 5% B. 8% C. 13% D. 25%

20. If 25% of the patients attending prenatal clinics in group B also attended the cardiac clinics, the number of prenatal clinic patients in group B who did NOT attend the cardiac clinics was MOST NEARLY

    A. 400 B. 450 C. 1200 D. 1350

21. If the number of persons who attended all clinics in group A last year was 20% less than this year, the number who attended the group A clinics last year was MOST NEARLY

    A. 32,700 B. 130,800 C. 163,500 D. 196,200

22. Assume that at the end of the year it was found that half of the people who attended the group B chest clinics had been found to be free of disease, 1/3 were discharged as needing no further care, and the rest were instructed to return to the clinic for further treatment.
    The number of persons who were told to return for further treatment was MOST NEARLY

    A. 7,000 B. 14,000 C. 21,000 D. 35,000

Questions 23-34.

DIRECTIONS: Each of Questions 23 through 34 consists of a word, in capitals, followed by four suggested meanings of the word. For each question, indicate in the space at the right the letter preceding the word which means MOST NEARLY the same as the word in capitals.

23. PUNCTUAL 23.____
    A. usual   B. hollow
    C. infrequent   D. on time

24. BENEFICIAL 24.____
    A. popular   B. forceful   C. helpful   D. necessary

25. TEMPORARY 25.____
    A. permanently   B. for a limited time
    C. at the same time   D. frequently

26. INQUIRE 26.____
    A. order   B. agree   C. ask   D. discharge

27. SUFFICIENT 27.____
    A. enough   B. inadequate
    C. thorough   D. capable

28. AMBULATORY 28.____
    A. bedridden   B. lefthanded
    C. walking   D. laboratory

29. DILATE 29.____
    A. enlarge   B. contract   C. revise   D. restrict

30. NUTRITIOUS 30.____
    A. protective   B. healthful
    C. fattening   D. nourishing

31. CONGENITAL 31.____
    A. with pleasure   B. defective
    C. likeable   D. existing from birth

32. ISOLATION 32.____
    A. sanitation   B. quarantine
    C. rudeness   D. exposure

33. SPASM 33.____
    A. splash   B. twitch   C. space   D. blow

34. HEMORRHAGE 34.____
    A. bleeding   B. ulcer
    C. hereditary disease   D. lack of blood

6 (#2)

Questions 35-40.

DIRECTIONS: Questions 35 through 40 are to be answered on the basis of the usual rules for alphabetical filing. For each question, indicate in the space at the right the letter preceding the name which should be filed THIRD in alphabetical order.

35. A. Hesselberg, Norman J.   B. Hesselman, Nathan B.   35. ___
     C. Hazel, Robert S.   D. Heintz, August J.

36. A. Oshins, Jerome   B. Ohsie, Marjorie   36. ___
     C. O'Shaugn, F.J.   D. O'Shea, Frances

37. A. Petrie, Joshua A.   B. Pendleton, Oscar   37. ___
     C. Pertweee, Joshua   D. Perkins, Warren G.

38. A. Morganstern, Alfred   B. Morganstern, Albert   38. ___
     C. Monroe, Mildred   D. Modesti, Ernest

39. A. More, Stewart   B. Moorhead, Jay   39. ___
     C. Moore, Benjamin   D. Moffat, Edith

40. A. Ramirez, Paul   B. Revere, Pauline   40. ___
     C. Ramos, Felix   D. Ramazotti, Angelo

Questions 41-50.

DIRECTIONS: Questions 41 through 50 are to be answered on the basis of the usual rules of filing. Column I lists the names of 10 clinic patients. Column II lists the headings of file drawers into which you are to place the records of these patients. For each question, indicate in the space at the right the letter preceding the heading of the file drawer in which the record should be filed.

COLUMN I		COLUMN II	
41. Charles Coughlin	A.	Cab-Cep	41. ___
42. Mary Carstairs	B.	Ceq-Cho	42. ___
43. Joseph Collin	C.	Chr-Coj	43. ___
44. Thomas Chelsey	D.	Cok-Czy	44. ___
45. Cedric Chalmers			45. ___
46. Mae Clarke			46. ___
47. Dora Copperhead			47. ___
48. Arnold Cohn			48. ___
49. Charlotte Crumboldt			49. ___
50. Frances Celine			50. ___

KEY (CORRECT ANSWERS)

1. D	11. A	21. B	31. D	41. D
2. B	12. C	22. A	32. B	42. A
3. A	13. B	23. D	33. B	43. D
4. D	14. C	24. C	34. A	44. B
5. C	15. D	25. B	35. A	45. B
6. D	16. D	26. C	36. D	46. C
7. B	17. B	27. A	37. C	47. D
8. B	18. A	28. C	38. B	48. C
9. C	19. C	29. A	39. B	49. D
10. A	20. D	30. D	40. C	50. A

EXAMINATION SECTION
TEST 1

DIRECTIONS: Each question or incomplete statement is followed by several suggested answers or completions. Select the one that BEST answers the question or completes the statement. *PRINT THE LETTER OF THE CORRECT ANSWER IN THE SPACE AT THE RIGHT.*

1. Of the following, the MOST important reason for requiring that an employee have knowledge of medical office procedures is that

    A. she can take care of sick people in the absence of a doctor
    B. patients in the clinic will be impressed with her apparent knowledge
    C. she will be more helpful in her work at the clinic
    D. letters she may have to write will be more concise

    1.____

2. A newly appointed employee should have a good understanding of her functions in the Department of Health.
Of the following, the training which would be LEAST helpful to her in the performance of her functions is

    A. an understanding of the role of the Department of Health in the community
    B. development of skill in the technics of work in a health center
    C. information as to the services offered in the health center
    D. development of skill in the care of the sick in their own homes

    2.____

3. If an employee were called upon at the same time to attend to each of the following, the one she should do FIRST is

    A. sterilize instruments used in the examination of the last patient
    B. answer the telephone
    C. give the patient who is just leaving another appointment
    D. check to see if a patient who has just arrived has an appointment

    3.____

4. Of the following, the LEAST important reason for answering telephone calls promptly in the health clinic is that

    A. patients waiting in the clinic will be impressed with the self-importance of the employee
    B. patients calling for information will be answered quickly
    C. the public will get a favorable impression of the Department of Health
    D. it will result in better service by keeping the lines free for other calls

    4.____

5. Assume that the physician assigned to the clinic in which you work calls the clinic and tells you that he has been detained for half an hour and will not be able to report at 1:00 P.M. as scheduled.
You should

    A. not say anything about the call to anyone
    B. report this information to your immediate supervisor
    C. tell the patient scheduled for 1:00 P.M. to come back the next day
    D. tell the physician that he must come at 1:00 P.M. since a patient has been scheduled for that time

    5.____

6. Assume that a physician who is examining a patient asks you to hand him a certain instrument from the tray. You do not know exactly what he is referring to.
   The BEST thing for you to do is to

   A. give him an instrument which you think might be suitable for the examination
   B. ask him to repeat what he said
   C. admit that you cannot identify the instrument he wants
   D. tell him that there is no such instrument on the tray

7. Assume that a patient asks you to explain something the doctor told her about her illness which she says she does not understand.
   For you to suggest that she tell the doctor that she did not understand what he told her and ask him to explain it again is

   A. *advisable;* the patient will be impressed by your interest in her
   B. *inadvisable;* patients get tired of the run-around
   C. *advisable;* the doctor is best qualified to answer questions concerning or affecting the patient's health
   D. *inadvisable;* the patient will lose confidence in your ability

8. Assume that, after you have been employed for several months, the nurse who is your immediate supervisor summons you to her office. She tells you that she has noticed on several occasions that you have been careless about your personal appearance. In this instance, it would be

   A. proper for you to tell her that your personal appearance is no concern of hers
   B. advisable for you to listen politely to her and then do nothing about it
   C. fitting for you to tell her that the other employees in the clinic are just as careless
   D. best for you to thank her for her interest and to tell her that you will make an effort to be more careful

9. One of the patients at the Health Center insists that she be sent to a different doctor as she does not like the doctor she saw last week.
   Of the following answers, the one that is MOST advisable for you to give to the patient is that

   A. she will have to take whatever doctor is available
   B. all the clinic doctors are equally good
   C. you will try to send her to another doctor
   D. she should see the nurse in charge

10. Suppose that the doctor in the clinic has given you an order which is contrary to the usual clinic procedure. Of the following, the BEST action for you to take is to

    A. point out to the doctor the usual clinic procedure and then do as he tells you
    B. refuse to do what he tells you as it is contrary to the usual procedure
    C. refuse to do what he tells you and call the nurse in charge
    D. do as the doctor tells you and at the first opportunity report the occurrence to the nurse in charge

11. When filing some patients' record cards in an alphabetic file, you notice that one card obviously has been misfiled.
    In this case, it would be MOST advisable for you to

    A. pay no attention to this as you believe it was not your error
    B. pull out the card and file it correctly
    C. report this to the clinic supervisor and suggest to her that she reprimand the employee who you believe is responsible for the misfiling
    D. take no particular care in the future when filing cards since errors will occur anyway

12. Assume that you are working directly with children in a well baby clinic. You feel feverish.
    Of the following, the BEST action for you to take is to

    A. wait and see whether you feel better; you don't want to seem to be a chronic complainer
    B. report immediately to the nurse in charge that you do not feel well
    C. take your temperature and, if it is over 101° F, report to the nurse in charge
    D. report to the nurse in charge only if you have other symptoms

13. As a receptionist in a public health center, you have certain responsibilities towards patients and other callers. You should greet each caller promptly and courteously. Never keep a caller waiting while you carry on a personal conversation, either on the telephone or with another employee. However, if you are occupied with clinic matters, give the caller to understand that you will be with him in a short while.
    On the basis of this paragraph, if a caller comes in while you are discussing with the nurse in charge coverage of the clinic during the lunch hour, the one of the following actions which would be the BEST for you to take is to

    A. stop and take care of his needs immediately as you should never keep a caller waiting
    B. nod to him and continue making plans for clinic coverage
    C. say to him that you will take care of him in a moment; then finish making your plans for clinic coverage
    D. finish making plans for clinic coverage with the nurse in charge and then inquire into the caller's needs

14. Assume that you are responsible for scheduling clinic appointments. One of the patients who has to report to the clinic every Tuesday morning asks that his appointments be scheduled for the last half hour of the clinic session. It has been the practice in this clinic to keep the last half hour open only for emergency appointments, and to schedule all appointments in order, from the time when the clinic opens.
    Of the following, the BEST action for you to take is to

    A. schedule the appointment at the time requested by the patient as he probably has a good reason for wanting it then
    B. disregard his request as no one attending a clinic should be given special consideration
    C. deny his request unless he has a medical reason for asking for a late appointment
    D. refer the request to the nurse in charge to determine if he should be given a late appointment

15. Suppose that a patient who is registered in the Social Hygiene Clinic of a Health Center appears in a drunken condition for a scheduled appointment.
Of the following, the BEST action for you to take is to

    A. inform the nurse in charge of the situation
    B. have him await his turn with the other patients
    C. send him home, telling him not to return until he is sober
    D. arrange for him to see the doctor immediately

16. Assume that you have been asked by your supervisor to instruct a newly-appointed aide in the performance of a given task.
Of the following, the BEST procedure for you to follow is

    A. to check her work only once after you have shown her how to do it; continued supervision after this should be the supervisor's responsibility
    B. not to check her work after you have shown her how to do it as she may resent your supervision
    C. not to check her work immediately but wait until she has done the task several times in order to give her a fair chance
    D. to check her work at frequent intervals after you have shown her how to do it until she is able to perform the given task

17. A worker should be carefully introduced to the clinic to which she has been assigned. The period of orientation will vary widely with the individual, her previous experience, and the type of clinic to which she is assigned.
In general, it will include an introduction to the physical set-up, the personnel, the type of service to be rendered, and the ideals of the clinic. In the beginning, the new worker should be given simple assignments and close supervision. The program should be arranged so as to give the nurse in charge opportunity to study the worker as to personality, general ability, or any special handicaps.
According to this paragraph, the one of the following statements that is MOST accurate is that, during the first few days, the new worker should

    A. do nothing but observe the physical set-up, the personnel, the type of service rendered, the ideals of the clinic
    B. be given a 30 hour course in the clinic to which she is assigned, including the physical set-up, the personnel, the ideals of the clinic
    C. be observed by the nurse in charge as to her ability to do the work in the clinic to which she has been assigned
    D. be closely supervised by the nurse in charge until she has a thorough knowledge of the clinic

18. Preparing a patient for physical examination has important mental aspects. Because each patient is individual in his reactions, a worker must plan her approach so as to deal with these reactions sympathetically. Thus, one patient may be afraid of the pain an examination may cause him immediately, another may fear that he will have unpleasant effects later, and still another may be only curious about the examination and have neither fear nor anxiety.
On the basis of this paragraph, the one of the following statements that BEST describes the reactions of patients when undergoing examination is that all patients

    A. are afraid when being examined
    B. react differently to an examination
    C. are afraid of the after-effects of an examination
    D. are curious about the examination

19. A recently published article states: Weight for height and age is, as many have previously held, an inadequate index of the *nutritional status* of a child. It is unscientific and unfair to set average weight as a goal for all children or for an individual child. Weighing and measuring, however, should be continued as a record of the trend of individual growth which is of value to the physician in relation to other findings and as valuable devices to interest the child in his growth.
According to this article, weighing and measuring the height of children

    A. are of no value and should be stopped
    B. are useful to the physician
    C. are of no value but give interesting information
    D. indicate the nutritional status of the child

19.____

20. Blood pressure is the force that the blood exerts against the walls of the vessels through which it flows. The blood pressure is commonly meant to be the pressure in the arteries. The pressure in the arteries varies with the contraction (work period) and the relaxation (rest period) of the heart. When the heart contracts, the blood in the arteries is at its greatest pressure. This is called the systolic pressure. When the heart relaxes, the blood in the arteries is at its lowest pressure. This is called the diastolic pressure. The difference between both pressures is called the pulse pressure.
The one of the following statements that is MOST accurate on the basis of this paragraph is that

    A. the blood in the arteries is at its greatest pressure during contraction
    B. systolic pressure measures the blood in the arteries when the heart is relaxed
    C. blood pressure is determined by obtaining the difference between systolic and diastolic pressure
    D. pulse pressure is the same as blood pressure

20.____

21. Lymph is a clear fluid, rich in white blood cells, and is actually blood plasma which has filtered through the walls of capillaries. It is circulated through the lymph vessels and in all the tissue spaces of the body. It carries nourishment and oxygen to the tissues and waste products away from them.
The one of the following statements that is NOT correct on the basis of this paragraph is that lymph

    A. contains red blood cells
    B. contains white blood cells
    C. is a basic part of blood
    D. is circulated through the body

21.____

22. When storing medical supplies, it is important to remember that liquids should be labeled

    A. only if the liquids are poisonous and there is the slightest chance that they will not be recognized
    B. whenever there is the slightest chance that they will not be recognized
    C. at all times, and discarded if labels have become detached
    D. only in those cases where the liquids will be given to patients

22.____

23. When dusting metal countertops in the clinic, it is BEST to use a clean cloth which is

    A. medicated   B. wet   C. dry   D. damp

23.____

24. Of the following statements concerning a hypodermic syringe, the one that is MOST correct is that a plunger

   A. used for taking blood specimens can be used with any syringe barrel
   B. can be used for any syringe barrel as long as it goes in easily
   C. can be used only with the syringe barrel that was made for it
   D. must be used with the syringe barrel that was made for it only if it is to be used for injections

25. The one of the following which should NOT be done when using a thermometer is to

   A. shake down the thermometer to 95F before taking the patient's temperature
   B. ask the patient to keep his lips closed when taking the temperature orally
   C. wash the thermometer in hot soapy water after use
   D. keep the thermometer in a container of alcohol when not in use

26. The temperature of an adult when taken by rectum is usually _____ than if taken _____ under the armpit.

   A. *higher;* either by mouth or
   B. *higher;* by mouth and lower than if taken
   C. *lower;* either by mouth or
   D. *lower;* by mouth and higher if taken

27. Of the following tests, the one which is associated with tuberculosis is the _____ test.

   A. Schick   B. Mantoux   C. Dick   D. Kahn

28. A needle that has been used to draw blood should be rinsed immediately after use in

   A. a disinfectant solution   B. hot water
   C. cold water   D. hot, soapy water

29. Of the following, the statement that is MOST correct is that a hypodermic needle should be checked for burrs, hooks, and sharpness

   A. once a week
   B. before it is sterilized
   C. after it has been sterilized
   D. after it has been used three or four times

30. The MOST accurate of the following statements is that, when a syringe and needle are being sterilized by boiling, the

   A. plunger must be completely out of the barrel
   B. needle should be left attached to the barrel as when in use
   C. plunger may be completely inside the barrel
   D. needle should be boiled at least twice as long as the syringe

31. Of the following, the MOST important reason for washing an instrument in hot soapy water is to

   A. sterilize the instrument
   B. destroy germs by heat
   C. destroy germs by coagulation
   D. remove foreign matter and bacteria

32. Assume that a hypodermic needle which is to be used for injection is accidentally brushed at the tip by your hand. Of the following, the action which should be taken before this needle is used is that it be

    A. washed under the hot water tap
    B. wiped with a sterile piece of gauze
    C. washed in hot soapy water, then rinsed in sterile water
    D. boiled for ten minutes

33. The CORRECT way to sterilize a scalpel is to

    A. place it in a chemical germicide
    B. boil it for 10 minutes
    C. put it in the autoclave
    D. pass it through a bright flame

34. Assume that a tray of instruments has been accidentally left uncovered for five minutes after it had been sterilized.
    Of the following, the action you should take to ensure that the instruments are sterile for use is to

    A. dip them in boiling water
    B. boil them for 10 minutes
    C. replace the cover on the tray
    D. wipe each instrument with sterile gauze

35. An intramuscular injection is MOST likely to be used in the administration of

    A. smallpox vaccine   B. streptomycin
    C. glucose   D. blood

36. The one of the following which is NOT a normal element of blood is

    A. hemoglobin   B. a leucocyte
    C. marrow   D. a platelet

37. Of the following statements regarding the Salk vaccine, the MOST accurate one is that it

    A. immunizes children and adults against paralytic poliomyelitis
    B. is a test to determine the presence of poliomyelitis virus in the blood
    C. is a test to determine whether a child is immune to poliomyelitis
    D. is used in the treatment of patients suffering from paralytic poliomyelitis

38. The GREATEST success in the treatment of cancer has been in cancer of the

    A. blood   B. stomach   C. liver   D. skin

39. An autopsy is a(n)

    A. type of blood test
    B. examination of tissue removed from a living organism
    C. examination of a human body after death
    D. test to determine the acidity of body fluids

40. The word *vascular* is MOST closely associated with

    A. the circulatory system
    B. respiration
    C. digestion
    D. the nervous system

41. The word *diagnosis* means MOST NEARLY

    A. preparation of a diagram
    B. determination of an illness
    C. medical examination of a patient
    D. written prescription

42. A tendon connects

    A. bone to bone
    B. muscle to bone
    C. muscle to muscle
    D. muscle to ligament

43. Blood takes on oxygen as it passes through the

    A. liver   B. heart   C. spleen   D. lungs

44. The fatty substance in the blood which is deposited in the artery walls and which is believed to cause hardening of the arteries is called

    A. amino acid   B. phenol   C. cholesterol   D. pectin

45. The digestive canal includes the

    A. stomach, small intestine, large intestine, and rectum
    B. stomach, larynx, large intestine, and rectum
    C. trachea, small intestine, large intestine, and rectum
    D. stomach, small intestine, large intestine, and abdominal cavity

46. When giving artificial respiration, it should be kept in mind that air is drawn into the lungs by the

    A. expansion of the chest cavity
    B. contraction of the chest cavity
    C. expansion of the lungs
    D. contraction of the lungs

47. The formula for converting degrees Centigrade to degrees Fahrenheit is as follows:

    Fahrenheit = 9/5 of Centigrade + 32°, or
    (multiply the number of degrees Centigrade by 9, divide by 5 and add 32)

    If the Centigrade thermometer reads 25°, the temperature, in degrees Fahrenheit, is

    A. 13   B. 45   C. 53   D. 77

48. To make a certain preparation, you have been told to mix one ounce of Liquid A and 3 ounces of Liquid B.
 If you have used 18 ounces of Liquid B in preparing a larger amount, the number of ounces of Liquid A you should use is

 A. 6   B. 15   C. 21   D. 54

49. If one inch is equal to approximately 2.5 centimeters, the number of inches in fifteen centimeters is MOST NEARLY

 A. 1.6   B. 6   C. 12.5   D. 37.5

Questions 50-52.

DIRECTIONS: Questions 50 through 52 are to be answered on the basis of the following situation.

you have been asked to keep records of the time spent with each patient by the doctors in the clinic where you are assigned, Iour notes show that Dr. Jones spent the following amount of time with each patient he examined on a certain day:

 Patient A - 14 minutes; Patient B - 13 minutes;
 Patient C - 34 minutes; Patient D - 48 minutes;
 Patient E - 26 minutes; Patient F - 20 minutes;
 Patient G - 25 minutes.

50. The average number of minutes spent by Dr. Jones with each patient is MOST NEARLY

 A. 20   B. 25   C. 30   D. 35

51. If Dr. Jones is to take care of the seven patients mentioned above at one session, the number of hours he will have to remain at the clinic is MOST NEARLY _____ hour(s).

 A. 1   B. 2   C. 3   D. 4

52. The one of the following groups of patients that required the LEAST time to be examined is Patients

 A. A, C, and E
 B. B, D, and F
 C. C, E, and G
 D. A, D, and G

Questions 53-60.

DIRECTIONS: Questions 53 through 60 are to be answered on the basis of the usual rules of filing. Column I lists the names of 8 clinic patients. Column II lists the headings of file drawers into which you are to place the records of these patients. In the space at the right, corresponding to the names in Column I, print the letter preceding the heading of the file drawer in which the record should be filed.

COLUMN I

53. Thomas Adams
54. Joseph Albert
55. Frank Anaster
56. Charles Abt
57. John Alfred
58. Louis Aron
59. Francis Amos
60. William Adler

COLUMN II

A. Aab-Abi
B. Abj-Ach
C. Aci-Aco
D. Acp-Ada
E. Adb-Afr
F. Afs-Ago
G. Agp-Ahz
H. Aia-Ako
I. Akp-Ald
J. Ale-Amo
K. Amp-Aor
L. Aos-Apr
M. Aps-Asi
N. Asj-Ati
O. Atj-Awz

53. _____
54. _____
55. _____
56. _____
57. _____
58. _____
59. _____
60. _____

KEY (CORRECT ANSWERS)

1.	C	16.	D	31.	D	46.	A
2.	D	17.	C	32.	D	47.	D
3.	B	18.	B	33.	A	48.	A
4.	A	19.	B	34.	B	49.	B
5.	B	20.	A	35.	B	50.	B
6.	C	21.	A	36.	C	51.	C
7.	C	22.	C	37.	A	52.	A
8.	D	23.	D	38.	D	53.	D
9.	D	24.	C	39.	C	54.	I
10.	A	25.	C	40.	A	55.	K
11.	B	26.	A	41.	B	56.	B
12.	B	27.	B	42.	B	57.	J
13.	C	28.	C	43.	D	58.	M
14.	D	29.	B	44.	C	59.	J
15.	A	30.	A	45.	A	60.	E

TEST 2

DIRECTIONS: Each question or incomplete statement is followed by several suggested answers or completions. Select the one that BEST answers the question or completes the statement. *PRINT THE LETTER OF THE CORRECT ANSWER IN THE SPACE AT THE RIGHT.*

Questions 1-6.

DIRECTIONS: In answering Questions 1 through 6, alphabetize the four names listed in each question; then print in the space at the right the four letters preceding the alphabetized names to show the CORRECT alphabetical arrangement of the four names.

1. A. Frank Adam B. Frank Aarons
   C. Frank Aaron D. Frank Adams
   1.____

2. A. Richard Lavine B. Richard Levine
   C. Edward Lawrence D. Edward Loraine
   2.____

3. A. G. Frank Adam B. Frank Adam
   C. Fanny Adam D. Franklin Adam
   3.____

4. A. George Cohn B. Richard Cohen
   C. Thomas Cohane D. George Cohan
   4.____

5. A. Paul Shultz B. Robert Schmid
   C. Joseph Schwartz D. Edward Schmidt
   5.____

6. A. Peter Consilazio B. Frank Consolezio
   C. Robert Consalizio D. Ella Consolizio
   6.____

Questions 7-13.

DIRECTIONS: For Questions 7 through 13, select the letter preceding the word which means MOST NEARLY the same as the word in capital letters.

7. LEGIBLE
   A. readable B. eligible C. learned D. lawful
   7.____

8. OBSERVE
   A. assist B. watch C. correct D. oppose
   8.____

9. HABITUAL
   A. punctual B. occasional
   C. usual D. actual
   9.____

10. CHRONOLOGICAL
    A. successive B. earlier
    C. later D. studious
    10.____

11. ARREST 11.____
    A. punish   B. run   C. threaten   D. stop

12. ABSTAIN 12.____
    A. refrain   B. indulge   C. discolor   D. spoil

13. TOXIC 13.____
    A. poisonous   B. decaying
    C. taxing   D. defective

14. TOLERATE 14.____
    A. fear   B. forgive   C. allow   D. despise

15. VENTILATE 15.____
    A. vacate   B. air   C. extricate   D. heat

16. SUPERIOR 16.____
    A. perfect   B. subordinate
    C. lower   D. higher

17. EXTREMITY 17.____
    A. extent   B. limb   C. illness   D. execution

18. DIVULGED 18.____
    A. unrefined   B. secreted
    C. revealed   D. divided

19. SIPHON 19.____
    A. drain   B. drink   C. compute   D. discard

20. EXPIRATION 20.____
    A. trip   B. demonstration
    C. examination   D. end

Questions 21-40.

DIRECTIONS: Column I lists 20 words, numbered 21 through 40, which are used in medical practice. Column II lists words or phrases which describe the words in Column I. In the space at the right, next to the number of each of the words in Column I, place the letter preceding the words or phrases in Column II which BEST describes the word in Column I.

COLUMN I	COLUMN II	
21. Anemia	A. A tube used to drain fluid from the bladder	21. _____
22. Anesthetic	B. The skull	22. _____
23. Arthritis	C. Inflammation of a joint	23. _____
24. Aseptic	D. A fluid injected into the rectum for the purpose of clearing out the bowels	24. _____
25. Astigmatism	E. A drug used in surgery which makes one insensible to pain	25. _____
26. Catheter	F. Rheumatic pain in the back	26. _____
27. Cranium	G. The branch of medicine concerned with diseases of the eye	27. _____
28. Diathermy	H. Examination of the inner parts of the body by use of x-rays and a special screen	28. _____
29. Enema	I. free from disease germs	29. _____
30. Electrocardiograph	J. Deficiency of blood	30. _____
31. Forceps	K. The branch of medicine concerned with diseases of women	31. _____
32. Gynecology	L. A tumorous growth	32. _____
	M. A structural defect of the eye	
33. Lesion	N. An apparatus for sterilization under pressurized steam	33. _____
34. Lumbago	O. The shoulder blade	34. _____
35. Microscope	P. A type of treatment which depends upon production of heat in the tissues by high frequency current	35. _____
36. Obstetrics		36. _____
37. Ophthalmology	Q. An instrument for recording electric changes caused by contraction of the muscles of the heart	37. _____
38. Postnatal		38. _____
39. Rabies	R. An instrument for magnifying minute organisms	39. _____
40. Stethoscope	S. The branch of medicine concerned with the care and delivery of pregnant women	40. _____
	T. A wound or injury	
	U. An acute infectious disease which is transmitted by the bite of dogs and other animals	
	V. A band of tissue which connects bones or holds organs in place	
	W. A medication used to calm nerves	
	X. An instrument used to listen to sounds in the heart	
	Y. A pair of tongs	
	Z. Occurring after birth	

KEY (CORRECT ANSWERS)

1.	C,B,A,D	11.	D	21.	J	31.	Y
2.	A,C,B,D	12.	A	22.	E	32.	K
3.	C,B,D,A	13.	A	23.	C	33.	T
4.	D,C,B,A	14.	C	24.	I	34.	F
5.	B,D,C,A	15.	B	25.	M	35.	R
6.	C,A,B,D	16.	D	26.	A	36.	S
7.	A	17.	B	27.	B	37.	G
8.	B	18.	C	28.	P	38.	Z
9.	C	19.	A	29.	D	39.	U
10.	A	20.	D	30.	Q	40.	X

EXAMINATION SECTION
TEST 1

DIRECTIONS: Each question or incomplete statement is followed by several suggested answers or completions. Select the one that BEST answers the question or completes the statement. *PRINT THE LETTER OF THE CORRECT ANSWER IN THE SPACE AT THE RIGHT.*

1. Keeping the tables and other surfaces clean in the examination room will help to break the _____ link in the chain of infection. 1.____

    A. portal of exit
    B. portal of entry
    C. mode of transmission
    D. reservoir

2. Of the following foods, _____ would typically serve as the best source of dietary fiber. 2.____

    A. kidney beans
    B. pears and apples
    C. lima beans
    D. celery

3. The identification of support resources available to a patient who wishes to enhance wellness would probably be included in the _____ stage of the nursing process. 3.____

    A. diagnosis
    B. evaluation
    C. planning
    D. implementation

4. According to the CDC, hand washing for the purpose of preventing the spread of microorganisms should be carried out for a minimum of 4.____

    A. 10 seconds
    B. 20 seconds
    C. 40 seconds
    D. 1 minute

5. _____ exercises are those that are designed to move each muscle and joint. 5.____

    A. Range of motion
    B. Rotation
    C. Isotonic
    D. Abduction

6. To establish and maintain therapeutic communication with an aphasic patient, a nurse assistant should 6.____

    A. familiarize the patient with ambient sounds
    B. ask simple questions that require "yes" or "no" answers
    C. speak slowly and enunciate clearly
    D. announce one's presence when entering the room

7. The nursing professional can make effective use of nonverbal cues to overcome

   A. a lack of understanding of cultural variations
   B. differences in values and beliefs
   C. cultural or language differences, such as mannerisms
   D. rapid information exchange with the hearing impaired

8. An early sign of vitamin C deficiency is

   A. eczema
   B. bleeding gums
   C. emaciation
   D. headaches

9. A patient needs to be repositioned in bed, but he is heavy. The nursing assistant is unsure about whether she can move the patient alone. The nursing assistant should

   A. seek the assistance of another nurse or nursing assistant
   B. wait until someone stronger comes on shift
   C. ask for the family's assistance
   D. move the patient as well as she is able

10. During a nursing assessment of a patient's nutritional status, the _____ serves as a measure of a patient's protein reserves.

    A. mid-upper arm circumference
    B. triceps skinfold
    C. subscapular skinfold
    D. body mass index

11. The _____ artery is used to measure blood pressure.

    A. brachial
    B. axillary
    C. radial
    D. ulnar

12. Of the following, strong body odor would most likely associated with

    A. sexual abuse
    B. physical abuse
    C. emotional abuse
    D. neglect

13. Each of the following is a tissue disease, EXCEPT

    A. Tetanus
    B. Strep throat
    C. Rheumatic fever
    D. Clostridium (gas gangrene)

14. On the diabetic exchange lists, which of the following would be the equivalent of one slice of bread?

    A. One bowl of cereal
    B. One baked potato
    C. 1/3 cup corn
    D. 1/2 glass milk

15. Which of the following illustrates the proper sequence for putting on PPE (personal protective equipment), from first to last?

    A. Mask, gloves, gown
    B. Mask, gown, gloves
    C. Gown, mask, gloves
    D. Gloves, gown, mask

16. Of the following nursing skills, _____ is most likely to be required during the pre-interaction phase of the nurse-patient relationship.

    A. a relaxed attending attitude
    B. decision-making
    C. recognizing limitations and seeking assistance
    D. empathy

17. A patient and a nurse are discussing the patient's physical activity levels and how they can be measured. Which of the following is NOT an appropriate measure of intensity?

    A. Pulse rate
    B. Talk test
    C. Rated perceived exertion (RPE) scale
    D. Perspiration amount

18. The sputum specimen comes from the

    A. lungs or bronchi
    B. pharynx
    C. nasal cavity
    D. oral cavity

19. The five stages of the nursing process, in their proper order, are

    A. Planning, Diagnosis, Assessment, Implementation and Evaluation.
    B. Planning, Diagnosis, Implementation, Assessment and Evaluation.
    C. Evaluation, Planning, Diagnosis, Implementation and Assessment.
    D. Assessment, Diagnosis, Planning, Implementation and Evaluation.

20. A patient's mail has been delivered to his room, but he hasn't noticed it. The nursing assistant should

    A. hand him the mail and offer to help as needed
    B. open the mail and ask if he would like the contents read
    C. make sure the mail doesn't contain anything that might be upsetting
    D. open the mail and leave it on the bedside table

21. Older and incontinent patients are generally more susceptible to urinary tract infections (UTIs), which involve the signs and symptoms of
    I. foul-smelling urine
    II. frequent urination
    III. painful urination
    IV. an inability to hold urine

    A. I and II
    B. I, II and IV
    C. II, III and IV
    D. I, II, III and IV

22. Which of the following is NOT a therapeutic communication technique?

    A. Offering opinions
    B. Reflecting
    C. Clarifying
    D. Stating observations

23. A nursing assistant who is making an occupied bed should

    A. raise the side rail on the unattended side
    B. place the dirty linen on the floor
    C. help the patient to sit in a chair while the bed is being made
    D. lower both side rails before removing the sheets

24. The Joint Commission on Accreditation of Healthcare Organizations (JCAHO) requires CDC guidelines for staff who care directly for patients who are at a high risk for acquiring infections. One of these requirements is that personnel should

    A. wear the full complement of PPE (personal protective equipment) during *every* patient encounter
    B. not wear artificial nails
    C. wear HEPA masks at all times
    D. not report to work if they have known contact with an infected person

25. A patient who is in restraints should have them moved and exercise his or her limbs every

    A. 45 minutes
    B. 2 hours
    C. 6 hours
    D. 12 hours

KEY (CORRECT ANSWERS)

1. D
2. A
3. C
4. A
5. A

6. B
7. C
8. B
9. A
10. A

11. A
12. D
13. B
14. C
15. B

16. C
17. D
18. A
19. D
20. A

21. B
22. A
23. A
24. B
25. B

TEST 2

DIRECTIONS: Each question or incomplete statement is followed by several suggested answers or completions. Select the one that BEST answers the question or completes the statement. *PRINT THE LETTER OF THE CORRECT ANSWER IN THE SPACE AT THE RIGHT.*

1. Among the body's nutrient reserves, _____ are most important to a person's resistance to infection. 1.____

    A. proteins
    B. carbohydrates
    C. fats
    D. vitamins

2. The CDC suggests that in order to produce health benefits, a person must engage in a level of physical activity that will allow them to expend _____ kilocalories per day. 2.____

    A. 80
    B. 150
    C. 250
    D. 400

3. In the planning phase of the nursing process for a patient at risk for pressure sore development, the major outcome is to 3.____

    A. maintain skin integrity
    B. regain intact skin
    C. regain ideal body weight
    D. demonstrate progressive wound healing

4. The Joint Commission on Accreditation of Healthcare Organizations (JCAHO) requires that the identification of patients be based on 4.____

    A. two separate identifiers for all services, not to include the patient's room number
    B. bar codes
    C. both the first and last name
    D. two nursing professionals double-checking all medications and procedures

5. A nurse must wear a gown to care for a patient in isolation. The nurse must 5.____

    A. not tie the gown, so it will be easier to remove later
    B. take the gown immediately to the dirty linen room afterward
    C. put the gown on after entering the room
    D. remove the gown before leaving the patient's room

6. A patient is recovering from a stroke, and the nursing assistant is helping the patient learn to walk again. The nursing assistant should 6.____

    A. encourage the use of a walker
    B. assist on the patient's weak side
    C. assist on the patient's strong side
    D. assist inconspicuously from behind

7. Symptoms of pneumonia include 7._____
   I. runny nose
   II. rapid pulse
   III. painful breathing
   IV. elevated body temperature

   A. I and III
   B. II and III
   C. II, III and IV
   D. I, II, III and IV

8. Each of the following is considered to be a "lifestyle" disease, EXCEPT 8._____

   A. cancer
   B. atherosclerosis
   C. typhus
   D. osteoporosis

9. Which of the following practices illustrates proper body mechanics for one who works in a health care facility? 9._____

   A. Picking up dropped objects by bending at the waist with back and knees straightened
   B. Standing upright, with the feet flat on the floor
   C. Lifting heavy objects by bending at the waist and using the muscles of the lower back
   D. Leaning into a patient when lifting him

10. Which of the following is a correct measure of urinary output? 10._____

    A. 12 oz
    B. 250 cc
    C. 1.2pt
    D. 1 1/3 cup

11. Analysis is a feature of the _____ of the nursing process. 11._____

    A. planning
    B. assessment
    C. diagnosis
    D. evaluation

12. The correct pulse range for an older adult is _____ beats per minute. 12._____

    A. 30-50
    B. 60-100
    C. 80-120
    D. 130-180

13. A(n) _____ can be used to assess the quality of nursing care while the care is being given.

    A. audit
    B. quality assurance review
    C. retrospective review
    D. concurrent review

14. The best approach to use with a patient who is having difficulty communicating verbally is to

    A. compose an assessment in the "multiple-choice" format
    B. be patient and provide verbal and nonverbal feedback
    C. ask the patient to write out any important information
    D. fall back on clinical language that can later be legally substantiated

15. The most obvious signs of prolonged immobility are usually manifested in the _____ system.

    A. musculoskeletal
    B. cardiovascular
    C. respiratory
    D. gastrointestinal

16. The primary sources of energy for the human body are

    A. minerals
    B. proteins
    C. carbohydrates
    D. fats

17. To provide a vegetarian patient with complete proteins, a nurse would combine in a single meal a portion of lentil soup and

    A. kidney beans
    B. milk
    C. whole wheat bread
    D. fish

18. Which of the following is NOT typically part of a nurse's physical fitness assessment?

    A. Skinfold measurements
    B. Joint flexibility
    C. Observing for signs of malnutrition
    D. Step test

19. A nursing assistant is using a waist restraint with a patient, under the physician's orders. The use of this restraint requires that the nursing assistant

    A. apply the restraint tightly enough to ensure non-movement
    B. release the restraint every couple of hours.
    C. watch closely for signs of skin irritation
    D. tie the restraint to the side rail

20. With a completely or partially immobilized patient, many nursing interventions for the respiratory system are aimed at promoting expansion of the chest and lungs. Which of the following would be most effective for this purpose?

    A. Aerobic exercise
    B. Frequent position changes
    C. Isometric exercises
    D. Physiotherapy

21. When entering the room of a patient who has tuberculosis, the nursing assistant wears a HEPA mask. The mask will protect the nursing assistant by breaking the _____ link in the chain of infection.

    A. susceptible host
    B. reservoir
    C. portal of entry
    D. portal of exit

22. When working with a hearing impaired resident, one should take care to

    A. speak in a normal tone of voice
    B. speak more loudly
    C. speak very slowly
    D. speak as little as possible

23. Cow's milk
    I. does not need to be boiled before being fed to infants
    II. is more easily digestible for an infant if it boiled than if it is pasteurized
    III. must be boiled over a direct flame for 2-3 minutes in order to be considered safe
    IV. should be pasteurized if it is going to be fed to an infant

    A. I only
    B. I and II
    C. II, III and IV
    D. III or IV

24. Of the following pathogens, the one that can have both harmful and beneficial effects is

    A. E. coli
    B. Giardia
    C. Staphylococcus
    D. Streptococcus

25. Which of the following areas will usually experience pressure when a patient is in the lateral position?

    A. genitalia (men)
    B. knees
    C. ilium
    D. vertebrae

KEY (CORRECT ANSWERS)

1. A
2. B
3. A
4. A
5. D
6. B
7. C
8. C
9. A
10. B

11. C
12. B
13. D
14. B
15. A
16. C
17. C
18. C
19. C
20. B

21. C
22. A
23. C
24. A
25. C

TEST 3

DIRECTIONS: Each question or incomplete statement is followed by several suggested answers or completions. Select the one that BEST answers the question or completes the statement. *PRINT THE LETTER OF THE CORRECT ANSWER IN THE SPACE AT THE RIGHT.*

1. The Heimlich maneuver is used for a patient who has

   A. a fresh wound that will not stop bleeding
   B. a blocked airway
   C. ventricular fibrillation
   D. trouble falling asleep

   1.____

2. Which of the following is NOT a major cause of fire in health care facilities?

   A. Paper or cloth piled in storage or patient areas
   B. Smoking by patients or staff in unauthorized areas
   C. Opening doors and windows for ventilation
   D. Faulty wiring or electrical equipment

   2.____

3. Which of the following is NOT a purpose of the medical chart?

   A. Reviewing patient care
   B. Directing patient care
   C. Recording patient response to care
   D. Disseminating information about patient care

   3.____

4. For a patient who has just finished bathing, a nursing assistant should wait a minimum of _____ before taking the blood pressure.

   A. 15 minutes   B. 30 minutes   C. 45 minutes   D. 1 hour

   4.____

5. Which of the following risk factors is MOST likely to be associated with falls?

   A. Angina
   B. Peripheral vascular disease
   C. Postural (orthostatic) hypotension
   D. Ventricular fibrillation

   5.____

6. Which of the following is an active strategy for health promotion?

   A. Immunization
   B. A low-fat diet
   C. Fluoridating a municipal water supply
   D. Fortifying homogenized milk with vitamin D

   6.____

7. A patient and a nurse are discussing the patient's physical activity regimen. The patient is interested in adding some strength training to her routine. One of the benefits of strength training is

   A. greater aerobic capacity   B. improved flexibility
   C. lower blood pressure   D. improved balance

   7.____

8. The basic nutrient required for tissue building and repair is

   A. vitamins
   B. carbohydrate
   C. fats
   D. protein

9. Generally, once a person reaches the age of _____, he or she is considered to be at risk for falls.

   A. 45
   B. 55
   C. 65
   D. 75

10. A nursing assistant is conducting an assessment of a patient's nutritional status. The typical diet history includes each of the following, EXCEPT

    A. height
    B. clinical signs of nutritional status
    C. the name of the person who usually prepares meals for patient
    D. personal crises

11. Medical asepsis

    A. renders an object free from all microorganisms
    B. is primarily a reactive measure to contamination
    C. involves handwashing before and after a medical procedure
    D. is unrelated to personal hygiene

12. The nursing care plan
    I. relates to the future
    II. focuses on actions designed to solve or minimize a problem
    III. is the product of a deliberate systematic process
    IV. is holistic in focus

    A. I and II
    B. I and III
    C. II and IV
    D. I, I, III and IV

13. The most effective and nonintrusive way to prevent dehydration of a patient is to

    A. install a saline drip
    B. offer fluids frequently while the patient is awake
    C. wake the patient frequently to offer fluids
    D. bathe the patient frequently

14. Each of the following is an element of body mechanics, EXCEPT

    A. alignment
    B. range of motion
    C. coordination
    D. balance

15. Signs and symptoms of insulin shock include each of the following, EXCEPT

    A. nausea
    B. dry, flushed skin
    C. fruity-smelling breath
    D. irritability

16. A nurse determines that a vegan patient needs to include iron-rich foods in her diet. Which of the following would best meet this requirement?

    A. Raisins
    B. Tuna
    C. Enriched pasta
    D. Molasses

17. One important limitation in applying Erickson's psychosocial development theory to nursing care is that it

    A. places an inordinate emphasis on sexual behaviors
    B. doesn't relate specific tasks to appropriate ages
    C. doesn't address cognitive or moral development
    D. does not consider the influences of biological factors

18. To avoid the buildup of static electricity in operating rooms, staff should avoid the use of

    A. long-sleeved gowns
    B. latex
    C. nylon
    D. spectacles

19. The planning phase of the nursing process would typically include

    A. discussing health care needs and priorities with the patient and family
    B. contacting other health resources
    C. discussing methods of implementation with the patient and family
    D. teaching therapies to the patient

20. Keeping a patient with a compromised immune system away from a carrier will help to block the _____ link in the chain of infection.

    A. portal of entry
    B. causative agent
    C. susceptible host
    D. mode of transmission

21. Which of the following food combinations would most likely correct a dietary iron deficiency?

    A. Cod liver and turnip greens
    B. Egg whites and beans
    C. Milk and oysters
    D. Whole wheat and apricots

22. Which of the following would NOT be an example of abuse or neglect?

    A. Leaving a patient in a soiled bed
    B. Restraining a patient according to a doctor's order
    C. Threatening to withhold meals
    D. Leaving a patient alone in a bathtub

23. A patient who is at risk for pressure sores would benefit substantially from each of the following dietary supplements, EXCEPT

    A. vitamin A
    B. vitamin C
    C. calories
    D. zinc

24. Parasympathetic responses to pain include

    A. nausea
    B. increased heart rate
    C. bronchial dilation
    D. dilation of pupils

25. General guidelines for turning a patient in bed include
    I. spread your feet at least 3 feet apart when lifting, to avoid injury to your own back
    II. roll the patient like a log to protect her spine
    III. if the whole body cannot be rolled at once, roll the legs first, then the upper body
    IV. pull or push whenever possible, rather than lift

    A. I only
    B. I, II and IV
    C. II and III
    D. I, II, III and IV

KEY (CORRECT ANSWERS)

1. B
2. C
3. D
4. A
5. C

6. B
7. D
8. D
9. C
10. B

11. C
12. D
13. B
14. B
15. D

16. A
17. C
18. C
19. C
20. C

21. D
22. B
23. A
24. A
25. B

———

EXAMINATION SECTION
TEST 1

DIRECTIONS: Each question or incomplete statement is followed by several suggested answers or completions. Select the one that BEST answers the question or completes the statement. *PRINT THE LETTER OF THE CORRECT ANSWER IN THE SPACE AT THE RIGHT.*

1. The most important natural barrier that helps people to prevent the entry of pathogens is 1.____

    A. mucus
    B. T cells
    C. cilia
    D. the skin

2. A patient has right-sided weakness. When dressing the patient in a blouse, the nursing assistant should 2.____

    A. put it on the right side first
    B. put it on the left side first
    C. pull it over the head and put both arms through at once
    D. put the right arm in a sling

3. Of the following, the activity most likely to be considered a secondary-prevention activity would be 3.____

    A. immunization
    B. preventing complications
    C. enhancing rehabilitation
    D. screening

4. Which of the following activities would generally burn the most kilo-calories per hour? 4.____

    A. Cross-country skiing
    B. Bicycling
    C. Canoeing
    D. Swimming

5. Which of the following is considered to be a kind of restraint? 5.____

    A. Gait belt
    B. Abductor wedge
    C. Posey vest
    D. Cannula

6. A patient has redness and clear drainage from her right eye. The medical abbreviation for right eye is 6.____

    A. O.D.
    B. R.E.
    C. O.S.
    D. E.R.

7. A nursing assistant has stored a disinfected batch of equipment in the supply closet. The disinfection would be invalidated by

   A. removing the equipment for use in another unit
   B. damage or water penetration of the packaging
   C. the movement of the equipment to another location in supply
   D. removing prepackaged items with ungloved hands

8. Direct nursing care is an element of the_____ stage of the nursing process.

   A. implementation
   B. assessment
   C. diagnosis
   D. evaluation

9. Vital signs include
   I. weight
   II. body temperature
   III. pulse rate
   IV. respiratory rate

   A. I and II
   B. I, II and III
   C. II, III and IV
   D. I, II, III and IV

10. A patient"s diet is found to be thiamin-deficient. Which of the following dietary elements would serve as the best remedy?

    A. Fruit
    B. Bread or cereal
    C. Beans
    D. Dairy products

11. Which of the following is NOT typically a physiological manifestation of stress?

    A. Pale skin
    B. Decreased urinary output
    C. Decreased blood sugar
    D. Dry mouth

12. A nursing assistant is preparing a patient for ambulation. Which of the following precautions is appropriate?

    A. Dressing the patient in clothing of his or her choosing
    B. Ensuring that the patient is not dizzy or disoriented
    C. Placing a towel over any spills on the floor
    D. Checking to see if the patient can stand alone before offering assistance

13. In the nursing process,_____ are stated goals for health care activities that can be used to plan and evaluate care.

    A. quality assurances
    B. audits
    C. standards of care
    D. criteria

14. A patient diagnosed with chronic pain may exhibit the defining characteristic of

    A. communication of pain descriptors
    B. altered muscle tone
    C. physical and social withdrawal
    D. guarded, protective behavior

15. The purpose of a turning sheet is to

    A. substitute for another person if nobody is available to move a helpless or heavy patient
    B. reduce friction when moving helpless or heavy patients
    C. serve as a light restraint while the patient's bed is being changed
    D. relieve pressure while supporting the patient's body

16. Of following patient positions, which typically promotes maximal chest expansion?

    A. Orthopneic
    B. Sims'
    C. Trendelenburg
    D. High Fowler's

17. Range of motion exercises can help
    I. increase aerobic capacity
    II. prevent contractures
    III. increase muscular strength
    IV. improve circulation

    A. I and II
    B. I and IV
    C. II, III and IV
    D. I, II, III and IV

18. _____ infections are associated with the delivery of health care services in a health care facility.

    A. Vector
    B. Nosocomial
    C. Exogenous
    D. Complementary

19. Each of the following is an appropriate action to take in caring for a patient with cancer, EXCEPT

   A. keeping the patient's skin clean, dry and pressure-free
   B. using surgical asepsis for infection control
   C. remaining positive and listening to the patient's concerns
   D. providing emotional support after hair loss

20. The FIRST stage of the nursing process is

   A. planning
   B. evaluation
   C. diagnosis
   D. assessment

21. Each of the following is typically involved in the nutritional assessment of a patient, EXCEPT

   A. measuring mid-upper arm circumference
   B. comparing weight to body build
   C. girth measurements
   D. a dietary history

22. Of the stages involved in death outlined by Elizabeth Kubler Ross, the last is usually

   A. acceptance
   B. depression
   C. denial
   D. anger

23. Of the following foods, _____ would most effectively boost the vitamin B content of a patient's diet.

   A. fruits
   B. dairy products
   C. simple sugars
   D. poultry

24. When changing unsterile dressing, the nursing assistant should wash hands
   I. before the procedure
   II. after removing the soiled dressing
   III. after the completion of the procedure

   A. I only
   B. II only
   C. II and III
   D. I, II and III

25. Which of the following would be a care consideration for maintaining the comfort of an elderly patient? 25.____

    A. Ensuing privacy
    B. Maintaining the patient's body temperature at a level that is agreeable
    C. Teaching about facility policies and procedures
    D. Allowing familiar caregivers access to the patient

KEY (CORRECT ANSWERS)

1.	D	11.	C
2.	A	12.	B
3.	D	13.	C
4.	A	14.	C
5.	C	15.	B
6.	A	16.	A
7.	B	17.	C
8.	A	18.	B
9.	C	19.	B
10.	B	20.	D

21.	C
22.	A
23.	D
24.	D
25.	B

TEST 2

DIRECTIONS: Each question or incomplete statement is followed by several suggested answers or completions. Select the one that BEST answers the question or completes the statement. *PRINT THE LETTER OF THE CORRECT ANSWER IN THE SPACE AT THE RIGHT.*

1. Which of the following positions is used specifically to relax tension of the patient's abdominal muscles?

    A. Knee-chest
    B. Trendelenburg
    C. Sim's
    D. Fowler's

    1.____

2. Approximately_____ percent of an average American's energy intake is derived from carbohydrates.

    A. 15
    B. 45
    C. 65
    D. 80

    2.____

3. When caring for a patient with a Foley catheter, it is important to

    A. remove the catheter for frequent inspection
    B. attach the drainage bag to the side rail of the bed
    C. empty the drainage bag at the beginning of every shift
    D. keep the drainage bag below the bladder

    3.____

4. The Joint Commission on Accreditation of Healthcare Organizations (JCAHO) requires that, in order to reduce the risk of falls, health care facilities such as hospitals should

    A. avoid prescribing medications that may contribute to falls
    B. educate patients about the dangers inherent in many medications
    C. establish a fall-reduction program and evaluate its effectiveness
    D. restrain patients who are at a high risk for falling

    4.____

5. Macronutrients include each of the following, EXCEPT

    A. carbohydrates
    B. fats
    C. proteins
    D. minerals

    5.____

6. A person's body temperature is
   I. lowest in the morning
   II. higher during infection in older patients than in younger patients
   III. highest in the afternoon or evening
   IV. most appropriately measured with a glass thermometer

   A. I only
   B. I and III
   C. II, III and IV
   D. I, II, III and IV

   6.____

7. A patient who is at risk for pressure sores should have a systematic skin inspection at least

   A. every 4 hours
   B. twice daily
   C. daily
   D. every 2 days

   7.____

8. A patient has experienced some hearing loss. In order to communicate clearly with the patient, a nurse should

   A. speak while looking directly at the patient
   B. use simple hand gestures
   C. speaking loudly and slowly
   D. speak in a higher pitch than normal

   8.____

9. A nursing assistant is teaching a patient how to perform range-of-motion exercises independently. He should instruct the patient to do each of the following, EXCEPT

   A. perform each exercise to the point of slight resistance
   B. perform each exercise three times
   C. vary the sequence of the exercises from day to day
   D. perform each series of exercises twice daily

   9.____

10. Which of the following is a method of cleaning equipment with chemicals or boiling water?

    A. Sterilization
    B. Disinfection
    C. Decontamination
    D. Antisepsis

    10.____

11. The best explanation for the relatively higher incidence of obesity in low-income communities is related to

    A. the food preferences of cultural or ethnic groups who predominate these populations
    B. a tendency to purchase greater amounts of pre-processed foods
    C. a greater reliance on daily products
    D. a reliance on cheaper cuts of meat

    11.____

12. The following steps to turning a patient from his back to his side in bed, in their proper order, are
    I. With your back straight and knees bent, pull the person toward you.
    II. Put both of your arms under the patient's waist and hips. Pull the hips toward you so the buttocks stick out a little.
    III. Put one arm under the patient's hips and the other under his up per back
    IV. Gently push to lift the hip and shoulder off the bed until the patient is resting on the hip and shoulder farthest from you.

    A. I, II, III, IV
    B. II, IV, III, I
    C. III, I, IV, II
    D. III, IV, I, II

13. A nurse is assessing a patient's ability to achieve wellness, applying the model of health promotion developed by Nola Pender. Which of the following would be considered a modifying factor involved in the patient's ability to participate in health-promoting behavior?

    A. The influence of the patient's family
    B. The patient's perceived level of control over his or her health
    C. The barriers that the patient perceives to health-promoting behavior
    D. The overall importance of health to the patient

14. The development of goals and objectives is an aspect of the _____ stage of the nursing process.

    A. assessment
    B. planning
    C. implementation
    D. evaluation

15. A patient is unresponsive. How many initial breaths should be administered before checking the pulse?

    A. 2
    B. 3
    C. 4
    D. 6

16. A patient is dying. The last sensory input she will lose will be her

    A. taste
    B. smell
    C. sight
    D. hearing

17. _____ precautions require the use of personal protective equipment within 3 feet of the patient

    A. Enteric
    B. Droplet
    C. Airborne
    D. Contact

18. Which of the following is the term for a sheet that is placed crosswise over the bottom sheet in the middle of a bed?

    A. Turning sheet
    B. Top sheet
    C. Drawsheet
    D. Transfer sheet

19. When transferring a patient, most of the patient's weight should be supported by the nursing assistant's

    A. shoulders
    B. upper arms
    C. legs
    D. back

20. A vaccination is an example of _____ health problem prevention.

    A. primary
    B. secondary
    C. tertiary
    D. prophylactic

21. A patient and a nurse are discussing the possibility of beginning a routine of moderate physical activity. The patient, who has been inactive for a long time, is concerned about the possibility of adverse effects. The most common adverse effect of physical activity is

    A. dizziness and anxiety
    B. cardiac arrest
    C. chronic fatigue
    D. musculoskeletal injury

22. If the diet of a child relies excessively on milk, the child is most at risk for a(n) _____ deficiency.

    A. calcium
    B. vitamin A
    C. vitamin D
    D. iron

23. When cleaning and disinfecting objects, nursing professionals should be led by each of the following guidelines, EXCEPT

    A. for the initial rinse, use hot water
    B. wash with hot water and soap
    C. for the final rinse, use warm water
    D. use an abrasive to clean equipment with grooves and corners

24. When treating a patient with pressure sores, the head of the bed should be elevated to a maximum angle of _____ degrees.

    A. 5
    B. 15
    C. 30
    D. 45

25. If a patient is isolated under enteric precautions, the purpose is usually to prevent

    A. infections transmitted by direct or indirect contact with infected blood or serae
    B. infections transmitted through direct or indirect contact with feces
    C. highly transmissible infections not requiring strict isolation but spread by close or direct contact
    D. stomach upset

KEY (CORRECT ANSWERS)

1.	D		11.	B
2.	B		12.	C
3.	D		13.	A
4.	C		14.	B
5.	D		15.	A
6.	B		16.	D
7.	C		17.	B
8.	A		18.	C
9.	C		19.	C
10.	B		20.	A

21. D
22. D
23. A
24. C
25. B

TEST 3

DIRECTIONS: Each question or incomplete statement is followed by several suggested answers or completions. Select the one that BEST answers the question or completes the statement. *PRINT THE LETTER OF THE CORRECT ANSWER IN THE SPACE AT THE RIGHT.*

1. The phrase "fifth vital sign" usually refers to

    A. blood glucose
    B. emotional distress
    C. functional status
    D. pain

2. Falls among elderly patients most commonly occur during activities that

    A. require physical dexterity
    B. are part of the person's daily routine
    C. involve high aerobic demands
    D. are risky and beyond the person's capabilities

3. A physician asks the nursing assistant to place a patient in the Sims' position. The patient should be

    A. in a semi-upright sitting position with the knees bent
    B. flat on the back with the head lower than the pelvis
    C. on her left side, left leg extended and right leg flexed
    D. in a kneeling position, supported by the knees and the shoulders, with the chest sagging down

4. Protective gloves should be used

    A. whenever one is within three feet of a patient
    B. only when directly handling specimens
    C. when there is actual, observable contact with blood or body fluids
    D. any time one is likely to touch a patient

5. The most common infecting organism associated with nosocomial infections is

    A. Enterococcus
    B. Staphylococcus aureus
    C. Lactobacillus
    D. E. coli

6. Each of the following is an important priority of data collection during the assessment stage of the nursing process, EXCEPT

    A. communicating with the patient, rather than consulting secondary sources
    B. including information about both strengths and needs
    C. arranging results in a way that is easily retrievable by future researchers
    D. including the patient's responses to current alterations

7. Signs of cerebrovascular problems include

   I. numbness
   II. blurred vision
   III. dizziness
   IV. shortness of breath

   A. I and II
   B. I, II, and III
   C. II and IV
   D. I, II, III and IV

8. The primary, secondary and tertiary levels of preventive action are elements of the_____ phase of the nursing process.

   A. assessment
   B. planning
   C. intervention
   D. evaluation

9. A patient is upset and crying about the recent death of his spouse. The most appropriate response to this would be to

   A. point out all the good things the patient can appreciate in his life
   B. leave the patient alone in his grief
   C. suggest some activities that might help the patient take his mind off things
   D. sit with the patient and allow him to talk about his feelings if he wishes

10. The performance of the Heinilich maneuver requires placement of the thumb

    A. just below the navel
    B. just above the navel
    C. right below the lower end of the sternum
    D. in the center of the sternum

11. A patient's dietary orders require that he receive a certain number of milliliters of juice. The container is a four ounce container. In order to determine the number of milliliters in the container, the nursing assistant should

    A. divide 30 by 4
    B. divide 60 by 4
    C. multiply 4 by 30
    D. multiply 4 by 60

12. A nursing assistant is putting a patient to bed for the night. Which of the following would NOT be a safety measure that should be taken?

    A. Using side rails
    B. Providing long intravenous tubing
    C. Using night-lights
    D. Placing the bed in a high position

13. At the primary level, health problem prevention is concerned with

    A. preventing the occurrence of health problems.
    B. discovering and treating existing health problems.
    C. easing the pain of existing, terminal health problems.
    D. reducing the severity of existing health problems.

14. "Nutrition" is most accurately defined as

    A. the kinds of food that a person habitually eats
    B. the sum of all the interactions between a person and the food he or she consumes
    C. the assimilation of food, through the stomach and bowels, into the body's organ systems
    D. the biochemical and physiologic processes by which the body grows and maintains itself

15. A nurse attempts to meet patient needs by applying Maslow's hierarchy to nursing care. In doing this, it is important for the health care professional to remember that the

    A. professional must always take modifying factors into account
    B. care should always focus on the patient's current needs, rather than strict adherence to the theoretical hierarchy
    C. hierarchy is not typically relevant to tertiary care
    D. patient's self-esteem needs must never be given priority over physiological needs

16. OSHA recommends that hypodermic needles should not be recapped if it can be avoided; however, if it is necessary, recapping should be performed using

    A. both hands
    B. at least one other person
    C. the one-handed "scoop" method
    D. puncture-proof gloves

17. Piaget's theory of cognitive development may be helpful to nurses in health promotion, in that it can help nurses to

    A. understand how children of various ages interpret health and health care
    B. identify the basic physical and psychosocial needs of children
    C. provide a basis for the assessment of a child's moral code
    D. provide a patient with tools to crisis-coping tools

18. To be sure that he is measuring a patient's weight accurately, a nursing assistant should weigh the patient

    A. at a different time each day
    B. after a meal
    C. after a nap
    D. at the same time every day

19. A patient and a nurse are discussing the patient's physical activity regimen. The patient wonders when would be the best time to perform stretching exercises. In order to increase flexibility, the best time to stretch is

    A. during moderate physical activity
    B. when checking the pulse
    C. during the post-exercise cool-down
    D. about an hour before exercising

20. The nursing assessment of a patient's nutritional status typically involves a dietary history of the patient's previous

    A. 24 hours
    B. 3 days
    C. week
    D. 2 weeks

21. A patient is deaf. The best way to communicate with her would be to

    A. use simple hand gestures
    B. speak loudly
    C. write out information
    D. speak slowly to allow for lip-reading

22. A nursing assistant is helping an immobilized patient to perform passive range-of-motion exercises. Which of the following would NOT be a guideline for this procedure?

    A. If contracture is present, the exercises should be stopped immediately.
    B. Body parts should be moved slowly. Move the body parts slowly
    C. Only the limb being exercised should be exposed.
    D. If rigidity occurs, pressure should be applied against the rigidity and the exercise slowly continued.

23. A nursing assistant has become annoyed with a patient's extreme depression and negativity, and is having a hard time viewing him objectively. In this situation, the most appropriate action would be to

    A. gently suggest that there are other patients in the same unit whose situations are more difficult
    B. excuse oneself and calm down outside the room, if doing so poses no risk to the patient
    C. confront the patient about the unhelpfulness of his attitude
    D. remind the patient that emotions and attitude can have a direct effect on one's health

24. The nursing history of an assessment that is concerned with infection risk will typically involve questioning the patient about each of the following, EXCEPT

    A. physical activity
    B. urinary frequency or difficulty
    C. appetite
    D. nausea

25. The CDC, to encourage greater participation in physical activity, recommends that people engage in a minimum of   25._____
    A. 60 minutes of high-intensity physical activity at least 3 days a week
    B. 60 minutes of moderate-intensity physical activity on most days of the week
    C. 30 minutes of moderate-intensity physical activity on most days of the week
    D. 30 minutes of light-intensity physical activity every day

---

KEY (CORRECT ANSWERS)

1. D
2. B
3. C
4. C
5. D

6. C
7. B
8. B
9. D
10. B

11. C
12. D
13. A
14. B
15. B

16. C
17. A
18. D
19. C
20. A

21. C
22. A
23. B
24. A
25. C

EXAMINATION SECTION
TEST 1

DIRECTIONS: Each question or incomplete statement is followed by several suggested answers or completions. Select the one that BEST answers the question or completes the statement. *PRINT THE LETTER OF THE CORRECT ANSWER IN THE SPACE AT THE RIGHT*

1. On a medical chart, the following phrase appears: "NPO until the return of peristalsis."
   This means the patient

   A. should eat soft foods only
   B. is on a clear liquid diet
   C. is on a full liquid diet
   D. is not permitted to eat or drink

   1.____

2. In epidemiology, the term "common vehicle" refers to

   A. an organism that carries a disease or infection to a human
   B. a living host for a pathogen
   C. the first link in the chain of infection
   D. material that has been contaminated and can transport pathogens

   2.____

3. When collecting data during the nursing process, a tertiary source of data would be

   A. the patient himself
   B. the medical record
   C. data from the patient's family and friends
   D. anecdotal observations

   3.____

4. Which of the following is a disinfecting agent?

   A. Povidone iodine
   B. Hibiclens
   C. Isopropyl alcohol
   D. Hydrogen peroxide

   4.____

5. Which of the following is most commonly the result of falls in the elderly?

   A. Vascular damage
   B. Gastrointestinal bleeding
   C. Soft tissue damage
   D. Hip fracture

   5.____

6. Generally, it is considered appropriate for a nurse or nursing assistant to share information regarding a patient's status with

   I. the staff on the next shift
   II. close family members
   III. the patient's roommate
   IV. other staff who do not have contact with the patient

   The CORRECT answer is:
   A. I only
   B. I or IV
   C. I, II or III
   D. I, II, III or IV

   6.____

7. Each of the following a factor that is likely to contribute to constipation, EXCEPT 7.____
   A. stress or anxiety
   B. decreased physical activity
   C. a low-roughage diet
   D. the routine use of enemas or laxatives

8. "Dangling" a patient serves to 8.____
   A. prevent foot drop
   B. give the attendant time to assume proper body mechanics before transferring
   C. acclimate him to the upright position
   D. assess orthostatic hypotension

9. A term that denotes total freedom from infection or infectious material is 9.____
   A. asepsis   B. disinfection
   C. quarantine   D. antisepsis

10. A patient has just finished a cold drink. Before taking an oral temperature, the nursing assistant should wait at least _____ minutes. 10.____
    A. 3 to 8   B. 10 to 20
    C. 30 to 45   D. 60 to 90

11. Which of the following would promote a patient's self-esteem while meeting social and mental health needs? 11.____
    A. Honest praise of the patient's accomplishments
    B. Letting the patient know that he is receiving the best care available
    C. Telling the patient that she is unique
    D. Accurate recording and reporting of observations

12. A statement of expected changes in a patient's health is called a/an 12.____
    A. objective   B. process objective
    C. outcome objective   D. goal

13. A patient has cognitive impairment and has trouble following instructions. A(n) _____ temperature should NOT be taken. 13.____
    A. tympanic (aural)   B. axillary
    C. rectal   D. oral

14. Which of the following nutrients is provided in significant quantities by eating fruits? 14.____
    A. Potassium   B. Niacin
    C. Phosphorus   D. Vitamin B

15. Nursing interventions for the completely or partially immobilized patient usually focus on

    A. achieving optimal elimination patterns
    B. restoring as much mobility as possible
    C. healing the syndrome or disease responsible for the patient's immobility
    D. preventing the hazards of immobility

15.____

16. Work practice controls in a health care setting are procedure that are designed to

    A. keep pathogens out of critical work areas
    B. achieve the repair or reprocessing of expensive protective barriers
    C. account for lost sharps
    D. reduce or eliminate the exposure to infection

16.____

17. The adaptive health model is focused primarily on the patient's

    A. stability   B. growth
    C. maturity   D. change

17.____

18. The most common method of assessing a patient's flexibility is to ask him or her to

    A. hyperextend the legs   B. perform several toe touches
    C. take a step test   D. perform two simple pull-ups

18.____

19. As an item of personal protective equipment (PPE), a mask will provide a protective barrier for about

    A. 10 minutes   B. 30 minutes
    C. 2 hours   D. 4 hours

19.____

20. The most significant sociological factor involved in community and family health is

    A. religion/spirituality   B. family size
    C. poverty   D. ethnicity

20.____

21 Which of the following is an important rule to remember when bathing a patient?

    A. Drain the tub immediately after the patient exits
    B. Allow the patient to be alone if he requests it
    C. Moisten any dry areas with bath oils
    D. Keep the call bell within reach

21.____

22. Which of the following is NOT a potential cardiovascular response to prolonged immobility?

    A. Thrombus formation   B. Venous vasodilation
    C. Postural hypertension   D. Diminished cardiac reserve

22.____

23. The basic level of the body's structure is the 23.____

    A. cell   B. organ
    C. system   D. tissue

24. In caring for a patient, a nursing assistant following Nola Fender's model of health promotion would direct her efforts toward 24.____

    A. determining the root causes of illness
    B. developing individual resources that enhance well-being
    C. assessing the strength of the patient's family
    D. limiting risk factors that impede wellness

25. A nursing assistant enters a patient's room to find him lying on the floor. The patient is conscious and responsive. The first thing the nursing assistant should do is 25.____

    A. ask the patient if he can sit on his own.
    B. check the patient for signs of injury
    C. help the patient up to a sitting position
    D. call for assistance from the supervising nurse

5 (#1)

KEY (CORRECT ANSWERS)

1. D
2. D
3. B
4. C
5. C

6. A
7. A
8. C
9. A
10. B

11. A
12. C
13. D
14. A
15. D

16. D
17. A
18. B
19. B
20. C

21. D
22. C
23. A
24. B
25. D

TEST 2

DIRECTIONS: Each question or incomplete statement is followed by several suggested answers or completions. Select the one that BEST answers the question or completes the statement. *PRINT THE LETTER OF THE CORRECT ANSWER IN THE SPACE AT THE RIGHT*

1. A family member has requested information about a patient. The most appropriate response would be to 1.____

    A. refer the family to the supervising nurse
    B. inform the family member about anything that is within one's scope of practice
    C. check with the patient first to seek approval for disclosure
    D. politely inform the family member that he is not entitled to this information

2. When using a gait belt to move a patient, one should 2.____

    A. tighten the belt while keeping two fingers between it and the patient's body
    B. tighten the belt while gripping it entirely in the fist of the other hand
    C. tighten it at the hips and then move it up to the waist
    D. allow the patient to tighten it to a point that is comfortable

3. When taking a patient's pulse, one observes each of the following, EXCEPT 3.____

    A. rhythm   B. force
    C. rate   D. pressure

4. The single most effective means for preventing the spread of infection is 4.____

    A. avoiding all contact with infected patients
    B. strict sterilization protocols
    C. PPE (personal protective equipment such as gowns, gloves, and masks)
    D. handwashing

5. Documentation is part of the _____ stage of the nursing process. 5.____

    A. assessment   B. planning
    C. implementation   D. evaluation

6. People with sleep problems are typically characterized by each of the following, EXCEPT 6.____

    A. listlessness   B. disorientation
    C. irritability   D. altered consciousness

7. Which of the following patient behaviors would be a sign of a partial airway blockage? 7.____

    A. Clutching the throat B. No movement of the chest
    C. Coughing   D. An inability to speak

8. Which of the following is considered a "modifying factor" in the health promotion model?

    A. Biological traits
    B. Perceived barriers to health-promoting behaviors
    C. Definition of health
    D. Perceived ability to control health

9. A nursing assistant wants to avoid pulling a male patient's catheter during turning. The catheter should be

    A. held in both the patient's hands during turning
    B. taped to the patient's upper thigh
    C. taped to the bed frame
    D. taped to the patient's hip

10. A patient presents the following clinical signs: muscle weakness and leg cramps, anorexia, nausea, and decreased bowel sounds. Most likely, the patient is suffering from a deficiency of the _____ ion.

    A. phosphate   B. potassium
    C. calcium   D. chloride

11. Which of the following hazards is unique to long-term care facilities?

    A. Spills
    B. Fire hazards
    C. Swinging doors
    D. Medications for chronic illnesses or disorders

12. Disinfection is a process that will generally kill each of the following types of organisms, EXCEPT

    A. bacterial endospores   B. protozoans
    C. bacteria   D. viruses

13. Of the following variables, is most significant in determining a person's total energy needs.

    A. age   B. physical activity
    C. immunity level   D. nutritional intake

14. Which of the following is a moist cold application?

    A. Ice collar   B. Disposable cold pack
    C. Ice bag   D. Cold compress

15. The formation of a hypothesis is an aspect of the _____ stage of the nursing process.

    A. assessment   B. planning
    C. implementation   D. evaluation

16. The correct way to remove a dirty isolation gown is to

    A. pull it off by the sleeve
    B. roll it dirty side in, away from one's body
    C. pull it over one's head
    D. let it drop to the floor and step out of it

17. A patient is a vegetarian who avoids all dairy products. Which of the following foods would typically serve as the best source of calcium for this patient?

    A. Okra
    B. Rhubarb
    C. Oranges
    D. Leafy greens

18. A nurse is evaluating a patient who has sustained a fall. The nursing evaluation should include a(n)

    A. orthostatic blood pressure
    B. complete minimum data set (MDS)
    C. PET scan
    D. flexibility test

19. The presence of a _____ increases the likelihood that a disease will occur in a particular person.

    A. risk factor
    B. mutation
    C. morbidity value
    D. relative risk

20. A patient's _____ temperature is generally most accurate.

    A. oral
    B. tympanic (aural)
    C. rectal
    D. axillary

21. Which of the following movements would be MOST likely to cause back injury?

    A. Rotation of the thoraco-lumbar spine
    B. Backward hyperextension of the spine, 20-30
    C. Lateral flexion of the quadratus lumborum
    D. Acute flexion of back with hips and knees flexed

22. At the secondary level, health problem prevention is concerned with

    A. discovering and treating existing health problems.
    B. preventing the occurrence of health problems.
    C. easing the pain of existing, terminal health problems.
    D. reducing the severity of existing health problems.

23. A nursing assistant placed clean bed linen in a patient's room, but the linen was not used. The bed linen should be

    A. used for the patient's roommate
    B. returned to the linen closet
    C. placed in the dirty linen container
    D. destroyed

24. Which of the following situations does NOT specifically require the use of antimicrobial soaps for handwashing by nursing professionals? 24.____

    A. Nurseries
    B. Before invasive procedures
    C. Recovery units
    D. When known multiple resistant bacteria are present

25. A nurse and a patient are working together to plan health promotion. Which of the following would they do FIRST? 25.____

    A. Assign priorities to behavior changes
    B. Identify effective reinforcements and rewards
    C. Develop a schedule for implementing behavior changes
    D. Determine barriers to change

KEY (CORRECT ANSWERS)

1. A
2. A
3. D
4. D
5. C

6. D
7. C
8. A
9. B
10. B

11. D
12. A
13. B
14. D
15. A

16. B
17. D
18. A
19. A
20. C

21. A
22. A
23. C
24. C
25. A

TEST 3

DIRECTIONS: Each question or incomplete statement is followed by several suggested answers or completions. Select the one that BEST answers the question or completes the statement. *PRINT THE LETTER OF THE CORRECT ANSWER IN THE SPACE AT THE RIGHT.*

1. Which of the following is a safety measure for a patient who is having a seizure? 1.____

   A. Moving the patient to a safer environment
   B. Placing something soft between the patient's teeth
   C. Restraining the patient
   D. Protecting the airway

2. To prevent pressure ulcers, an immobilized patient should be repositioned 2.____

   A. hourly
   B. every 2 hours
   C. every 4 hours
   D. twice daily

3. Which of the following is NOT an appropriate fall prevention strategy? 3.____

   A. Monitoring patient for vital sign changes
   B. Restraining the patient
   C. Educating the patient about fall risks
   D. Safety checks for home environmental hazards

4. The level of aseptic control that destroys all pathogens is 4.____

   A. disinfection
   B. sanitation
   C. decontamination
   D. sterilization

5. Gloves MUST be worn when 5.____

   A. assisting in range of motion exercises
   B. giving a sponge bath
   C. performing perineal care
   D. feeding a patient

6. Of the following, a(n) _____ patient is LEAST likely to have a decubitus ulcer. 6.____

   A. incontinent
   B. overweight
   C. immobile
   D. post-surgical

7. Data collection and analysis are aspects of the _____ stage of the nursing process. 7.____

   A. assessment
   B. planning
   C. diagnosis
   D. evaluation

8. The state of sleep is NOT typically characterized by 8.____

   A. decreased responsiveness to external stimuli
   B. minimal or no change in the body's physiologic processes
   C. variable levels of consciousness
   D. minimal physical activity

9. The earliest sign of a pressure sore is

   A. numbness
   B. clamminess
   C. swelling
   D. discoloration

10. Micronutrients include

    A. fats
    B. vitamins
    C. proteins
    D. carbohydrates

11. Parasympathetic responses to pain include

    A. diaphoresis
    B. variable breathing patterns
    C. pallor
    D. increased pulse rate

12. Which of the following safety devices would be used to transfer a dependent patient from a bed to a chair?

    A. Quad cane
    B. Gait belt
    C. Posey vest
    D. EasyStand

13. Each of the following is an example of primary illness prevention, EXCEPT

    A. immunization
    B. teaching breast self-examination
    C. family planning services
    D. environmental sanitation

14. Patients with a one-sided weakness would use _____ for ambulation.

    A. a walker
    B. a cane
    C. crutches
    D. a wheelchair

15. When making strenuous movements, a partially immobilized patient tends to force expiration against a closed airway. This activity is known as

    A. the Heimlich maneuver
    B. Korotkoff sounding
    C. apnea
    D. the Valsalva maneuver

16. Erickson's theory of psychosocial development states that from ages one to three, the toddler's primary task is to develop

    A. trust
    B. ingenuity
    C. autonomy
    D. self-concept

17. Instruments that are used to invade a patient's nonsterile body sites must undergo

    A. high-level disinfection
    B. sanitation
    C. decontamination
    D. sterilization

18. Wheelchairs, beds, and stretchers should be locked   18.____
    A. whenever a patient is being positioned or moved
    B. when the clear possibility of a fall is evident
    C. only when requested by the patient or a family member
    D. only when the patient will be in the wheelchair, bed, or stretcher for an extended period

19. According to Maslow's hierarchy of needs, the types of needs are considered most basic to a person's health are   19.____
    A. physiological   B. self-esteem
    C. love and belonging   D. safety and security

20. The process of restoring a disabled patient to the highest possible level of functioning is known as   20.____
    A. rejuvenation   B. restoration
    C. remission   D. rehabilitation

21. As the nursing process method first came into accepted use, most practitioners' attention was focused on   21.____
    A. diagnosis   B. assessment
    C. evaluation   D. implementation

22. What is the term used to describe a person's ability to share or understand another person's feelings?   22.____
    A. Clairvoyance   B. Sympathy
    C. Empathy   D. Pity

23. Which of the following foods would NOT be included in a clear liquid diet?   23.____
    A. Sherbet   B. Hard candy
    C. Broth   D. Gelatin

24. The most commonly measured pulse is the _____ pulse.   24.____
    A. ulnar   B. brachial
    C. radial   D. carotid

25. In general, a patient at risk for impaired skin integrity should perform active range-of-motion exercises every   25.____
    A. hour   B. 2-3 hours
    C. 4-6 hours   D. day

KEY (CORRECT ANSWERS)

1.	D	11.	B
2.	B	12.	B
3.	B	13.	B
4.	D	14.	B
5.	C	15.	D
6.	D	16.	C
7.	A	17.	A
8.	B	18.	A
9.	D	19.	A
10.	B	20.	D

21. B
22. C
23. A
24. C
25. B

EXAMINATION SECTION
TEST 1

DIRECTIONS: Each question or incomplete statement is followed by several suggested answers or completions. Select the one that BEST answers the question or completes the statement. *PRINT THE LETTER OF THE CORRECT ANSWER IN THE SPACE AT THE RIGHT.*

1. Those who are legally entitled to view a client's medical records without written consent include
    I. health care professionals who are caring for the client
    II. the client's insurer
    III. the client's son or daughter
    IV. the client's immediate nuclear family

    A. I only
    B. I and II
    C. I, II and III
    D. I, II, III and IV

2. For a nurse who provides community-based services in a senior center populated mostly by Asian-American clients, the most important preparatory skill or ability would be

    A. specialized knowledge in geriatric care
    B. mastery of how the health-care system works
    C. knowledge of the clients' culture
    D. knowledge of nutrition

3. Which of the following is an important source of insoluble dietary fiber?

    A. Whole grain foods
    B. Sweet potatoes
    C. Oats
    D. Soybeans

4. Factors that are known to contribute to heart disease include each of the following, EXCEPT

    A. sedentary lifestyle
    B. diabetes mellitus
    C. hyperlipidemia
    D. low triglycerides

5. _____ is a physiological process that affects oxygenation by limiting the amount of inspired oxygen that is delivered to the alveoli.

    A. Anemia
    B. Bradycardia
    C. Airway obstruction
    D. Fever

6. Which of the following types of data, collected during the assessment phase, would be considered subjective?

    A. The client's temperature is 98.
    B. The nurse observes that the client's face is flushed.
    C. The client states that he is nauseated and thirsty.
    D. The client's pulse is 100.

7. A nurse is designing a client teaching program that makes use of the humanistic model. The nurse's program is aimed at the client goal of

    A. becoming able to establish and maintain lifelong intimate relationships
    B. achieving her full potential
    C. gaining insight into her own behavior and being able to modify it
    D. becoming a productive member of society

8. Typically, a client's mental status is MOST effectively assessed by

    A. observing the client during the interview and examination
    B. having the client describe her mental status
    C. observing responses to a list of questions prepared in advance
    D. observing reactions to provocative questions

9. Nurses use critical thinking in the daily practice of nursing by

    A. anticipating likely medical diagnoses
    B. ensuring that there are adequate supplies on hand
    C. making conversions during medication dosage calculations
    D. setting priorities for the day

10. The oxygenation rate within body cells is regulated by the _____ gland.

    A. adrenal
    B. pineal
    C. thyroid
    D. apocrine

11. A nurse leads a group discussion on nutrition, and then asks the participants to decide on a topic of discussion for the next meeting. The nurse is representing the _____ leadership style.

    A. autocratic
    B. democratic
    C. exploitive
    D. laissez-faire

12. In order to be functional and appropriate for the situation, the nurse-client relationship must be

    A. established in an early stage by means of the nurse's statement of purpose
    B. developed from joint problem-solving work between nurse and client
    C. open-ended
    D. established by the client's willingness to accept the nurse's interventions

13. A client in a full arm cast expresses concern about preventing atrophy of the muscles in his upper arm. Assuming exercise is not contraindicated, the nurse should recommend _____ exercises.

    A. weightlifting
    B. kinetic
    C. aerobic
    D. isometric

14. An elderly client who lives at home has a history of glaucoma, for which she takes drops daily. She reports a loss of peripheral vision and an inability to adjust to darkness. Which of the following nursing diagnoses is most appropriate for her?

    A. High risk of injury related to sensory deficit
    B. High risk of injury related to impaired verbal communication
    C. High risk of injury related to lack of home safety precautions
    D. High risk for poisoning related to inadequate safeguards on medication

15. The presence of hyperemia represents the _____ stage of the inflammatory response.

    A. resolution
    B. granuloma
    C. acute vascular response
    D. chronic cellular response

16. During an assessment interview, the nurse should
    I. ask about the main problem first
    II. focus on the client, and not the signs or symptoms
    III. rely mostly on direct questions
    IV. try to avoid commentary unless it is absolutely necessary

    A. I and II
    B. I, II and IV
    C. II and III
    D. I, II, III and IV

17. Of the following clients, which would LEAST likely suffer from an imbalance in fluid, acid-base, or electrolytes?

    A. An adult with impaired cardiac function
    B. An elderly client with dementia
    C. A middle-aged client suffering from a Stage II pressure ulcer
    D. A two-year-old that has had gastroenteritis for four days

18. An overweight client with gout is discussing his diet with the nurse. During their discussion, the client should demonstrate an understanding of which foods have a high purine content. Which of the following foods would be MOST appropriate for this client?

    A. Liver
    B. Broccoli
    C. Lentils
    D. Wheat bran

19. A client has been diagnosed with terminal cancer. Shortly after the diagnosis she turns to the nurse and asks: "What should I do?" The nurse responds: "What do you think would be best for you and your family?"
    The nurse has used the therapeutic communication technique of

    A. Acknowledging
    B. Refraining
    C. Metacommunication
    D. Reflecting

20. Which of the following is NOT considered a task involved in the orientation phase of the nurse-client relationship?

    A. Exploring the client's thoughts and feelings
    B. Exploring one's own feelings and fears
    C. Clarifying the problem
    D. Structuring and developing the contract

21. One of the first clinical signs of hypovolemia associated with fluid volume deficit is

    A. tachycardia
    B. edema
    C. bradycardia
    D. shortness of breath

22. A nurse is asked to obtain an arterial blood gas from a client. Of the following, the _____ artery is the LEAST appropriate site for obtaining the blood sample.

    A. femoral
    B. brachial
    C. subclavian
    D. radial

23. Parasthesia is a condition that may in itself become the etiology for other nursing diagnoses, such as

    A. knowledge deficit
    B. fibromyalgia
    C. dehydration
    D. risk for injury

24. A client diagnosed with acute pain may exhibit the defining characteristic of

    A. weight change
    B. sympathetic nervous system responses
    C. depression
    D. sleep pattern changes

25. A food label contains the following information: 25.____
    2 grams of protein
    12 grams of fat
    15.5 grams of carbohydrate
    Using the 4-4-9 method, the nurse calculates the number of total calories to be

    A. 36
    B. 97
    C. 178
    D. 256

KEY (CORRECT ANSWERS)

1. A
2. C
3. A
4. D
5. C

6. C
7. B
8. A
9. D
10. C

11. B
12. B
13. D
14. A
15. C

16. B
17. C
18. B
19. D
20. B

21. A
22. C
23. D
24. B
25. C

TEST 2

DIRECTIONS: Each question or incomplete statement is followed by several suggested answers or completions. Select the one that BEST answers the question or completes the statement. *PRINT THE LETTER OF THE CORRECT ANSWER IN THE SPACE AT THE RIGHT.*

1. Which of the following is an example of palliative surgery?   1.____

    A. Vascular grafting
    B. Nephrectomy
    C. Laparatomy
    D. Nerve block

2. A client has a respiratory disease that causes a chronic lack of oxygen. The nurse would need to expect and be most watchful for   2.____

    A. peripheral edema
    B. wheezing upon exhaling
    C. flushed skin
    D. clubbing of the digits

3. In reviewing the file of a client who is scheduled for an IV pyelogram, which of the following should receive the nurse's special attention?   3.____

    A. Hypertension
    B. Iodine allergy
    C. Diabetes mellitus
    D. Latest bowel movement

4. Which of following is NOT an advantage associated with the use of closed questions in interviewing a client?   4.____

    A. Greater potential for revealing a client's emotional state
    B. Ease of documentation
    C. Less skill required of the interviewer
    D. More effective control of answers

5. Of the possible complications associated with blood transfusion, the most serious is   5.____

    A. allergic reaction
    B. fever
    C. hemolysis
    D. dizziness

6. Which of the following cranial nerves is NOT assessed by evaluating the eyes and vision?   6.____

    A. First
    B. Third
    C. Fifth
    D. Sixth

7. A 78-year-old client is brought to the emergency department after suffering vomiting and diarrhea for the last 48 hours. During the nursing assessment, the nurse observes that the client's skin is dry and can be tented, and that the client complains of an itching sensation. In developing a plan of care for the client, the most appropriate diagnosis would be

   A. risk for fall related to sensory deficit, as manifested by prolonged diarrhea and vomiting
   B. risk for fluid volume deficit related to prolonged diarrhea and vomiting
   C. risk for fluid volume excess related to prolonged diarrhea and vomiting
   D. nutrition imbalanced: less than body requirements, related to prolonged diarrhea and vomiting

8. A client who is several days post-surgery complains that none of his family has been to see him since the operation. The nurse responds: "That was your son who was here just this morning, wasn't it—The man who brought those flowers?"
   The type of therapeutic communication technique being used by the nurse is

   A. reflection
   B. focusing
   C. clarifying
   D. confrontation

9. Each of the following is a factor that commonly contributes to constipation, EXCEPT

   A. anxiety or stress
   B. decreased activity level
   C. low dietary fiber
   D. routine use of laxatives

10. The most significant contributing factor in cardiac disease is

    A. hypotension
    B. congenital heart defects
    C. alcohol abuse
    D. atherosclerosis

11. Clients are often encouraged to perform deep breathing exercises after surgery, in order to

    A. counteract respiratory acidosis
    B. increase cardiac output
    C. expand residual volume
    D. increase blood volume

12. Which of the following hormones acts to preserve sodium ions in the body's cells?

    A. Thyrocalcitonin
    B. Androstenone
    C. Cortisone
    D. Aldosterone

13. Which of the following is NOT an example of tertiary care?

    A. Neurosurgery
    B. Promoting workplace safety
    C. Hospice care
    D. Burn care

14. A client has died. Because proper handling of a client's body after death is an important intervention, the nurse should

    A. cover the client completely with a sheet before family members are allowed into the room
    B. apply makeup, jewelry, and any other accessories that the person wore in life before allowing the family into the room
    C. make sure the body looks as clean and natural as possible
    D. leave the body exactly as it was at the moment of death until a physician has arrived to formalize the death pronouncement

15. The nurse is meeting a new client. Which of the following would be MOST effective in initiating the nurse-client relationship?

    A. Asking the client why she was brought to the hospital.
    B. Explaining the purpose of and plan for the relationship
    C. Waiting until the client indicates a readiness to establish a relationship.
    D. Describing her family background, and then asking the client to do the same.

16. Together, a nurse and a client devise a nursing care plan with one goal being the maintenance of adequate fluid volume. The achievement of this goal can most accurately be measured by

    A. auscultation for heart and vascular sounds
    B. palpating for skin turgor, pulse, and heart rhythm
    C. monitoring bowel elimination patterns
    D. monitoring serum glucose

17. Nursing care and treatment of pressure sores is executed under each of the following general guidelines or recommended practices, EXCEPT the

    A. use of alcohol to clean and dress sores
    B. frequent repositioning of the client
    C. tissue sampling from infected sores
    D. application of cornstarch to the bedsheet

18. Clients should be screened for tuberculosis every

    A. six months
    B. year
    C. 2 years
    D. 5 years

19. Which of the following represents a primary source of data during the assessment phase of the nursing process?

    A. The client states that she has been suffering from intermittent dizzy spells.
    B. The client's spouse says the she has seemed severely fatigued lately.
    C. The client's chart documents a history of epilepsy.
    D. The client's temperature is 99° F.

20. A client with a broken left hand is awaiting an X-ray. Which of the following nonpharmacological interventions is most appropriate to help the client reduce pain prior to the procedure?

    A. Applying ice directly over the break
    B. Turning of the lights and eliminating other sensory stimuli
    C. Applying ice to the left elbow
    D. Applying warmth directly over the break

21. A nurse is planning an educational program on the detection of cancer, to be presented at a community clinic. Which of the following elements is LEAST likely to help address the various learning styles of the clients?

    A. A lecture
    B. Specific examples/case studies
    C. Audiovisuals
    D. Collaborative activities

22. Which of the following is an example of an outcome evaluation?

    A. A review of nursing documentation for compliance with institutional standards
    B. A survey to analyze staffing patterns
    C. Checking a client's temperature before administering a new medication
    D. An audit that records the number of postoperative infections

23. Which of the following tasks is part of the working phase of the nurse-client relationship?

    A. Identifying client problems
    B. Establishing trust
    C. Developing a plan for interaction
    D. Reviewing progress and attainment of goals

24. Which of the following is the body's mechanism for preventing pressure sores?

    A. third-space movement
    B. ischemia
    C. vasoconstriction
    D. vasodilation/hyperemia

25. If a client is hearing-impaired, the nurse should establish and maintain therapeutic communication by

    A. learning sign language
    B. using an inteipreter
    C. using simple sentences
    D. orienting the client to sounds in the environment

KEY (CORRECT ANSWERS)

1. D
2. D
3. B
4. A
5. C

6. A
7. B
8. C
9. A
10. D

11. A
12. D
13. B
14. C
15. A

16. B
17. A
18. C
19. A
20. C

21. A
22. D
23. A
24. D
25. C

TEST 3

DIRECTIONS: Each question or incomplete statement is followed by several suggested answers or completions. Select the one that BEST answers the question or completes the statement. *PRINT THE LETTER OF THE CORRECT ANSWER IN THE SPACE AT THE RIGHT.*

1. A nurse asks a client: "What kind of abdominal pain are you feeling today?" What kind of assessment is being performed? 1.____

    A. Time-lapsed
    B. Problem-focused
    C. Initial
    D. Emergency

2. A client has been placed on a high-fiber diet. Which of the following foods would be LEAST likely to contribute to the diet? 2.____

    A. Green peppers
    B. Cheese
    C. Apples
    D. Wheat bread

3. A "chronic" illness is generally defined as one that lasts for more than 3.____

    A. six weeks
    B. 3 months
    C. 6 months
    D. 1 year

4. Which of the following is NOT a sign of cardiac arrest? 4.____

    A. Crepitations auscultated in lungs
    B. No carotid pulse
    C. Dilated pupils
    D. Apnea

5. For a client who is admitted with gastrointestinal bleeding, one of the earliest and most important blood tests will be the 5.____

    A. complete blood count
    B. Coombs test
    C. arterial blood gases
    D. lipid panel

6. A nursing care plan for a client with a diagnosis of chronic pain related to compression of the spinal nerves involves two goals: the client will achieve a sense of pain relief within 1 month, and the client will perform self-care measures with less discomfort on self-report within 14 days. Which of the following would be an appropriate evaluation of the effectiveness of the care plan? 6.____

    A. Observing whether client has returned to social activities within 14 days
    B. Observing the client's facial expression in response to the application of localized heat
    C. Observing client's freedom of movement and facial expressions for signs of discomfort
    D. Asking if client's pain has remained localized within initially described boundaries

7. In planning client teaching, the nurse's instruction should be most significantly guided by the knowledge that

   A. each client has unique learning needs
   B. a client's cultural background is the most important factor in determining his or her learning needs
   C. all clients share the same basic learning needs
   D. a client's learning needs are most strongly correlated with his or her life stage

8. One of the goals of a nursing care plan is for a client to return to within 10 percent of his ideal body weight. Each of the following would be an appropriate outcome to go along with this goal, EXCEPT

   A. the client loses 2 kg per week
   B. the client gains 2 kg per week
   C. the client verbalizes positive feelings about weight loss or gain
   D. the client selects appropriate foods to facilitate weight gain or loss

9. A client is recovering from a stroke and is aphasic. To establish and maintain therapeutic communication with this client, the nurse should

   A. ask brief questions that require "yes" or "no" answers
   B. be sure to provide some introductory language before each procedure or activity
   C. make as many decisions as feasible for the client, to avoid agitating her
   D. speak very slowly and enunciate clearly

10. A client is semiconscious and likely to obstruct her own airway with her tongue. If the client requires respiratory intubation and there are no contraindications, a(n) _____ tube should be used.

    A. oropharyngeal
    B. endotracheal
    C. tracheostomy
    D. nasopharyngeal

11. A nurse asks a client to close his eyes, and then places a spoon in his palm and asks the client to identify the object. Which evaluation is the nurse performing?

    A. Stereognosis
    B. Tactile spatial acuity
    C. Texture discrimination
    D. Proprioception

12. A 38-year-old woman has a diagnosis of nocturia, probably caused by pregnancy. The nurse should recommend that the client

    A. restrict fluid intake in evening and nighttime hours
    B. consult a urologist
    C. make use of a nighttime alarm to alert her when an episode is occurring
    D. avoid eating citrus fruits

13. A doctor has ordered that a client take 6 ml of a medication in solution. The nurse's equipment is marked for fluid ounces (oz). How many ounces should the nurse administer?

    A. 0.2
    B. 0.8
    C. 1.2
    D. 2.4

14. A nurse is assessing a new client for possible impairment of verbal communication. Each of the following should be a component of the assessment, EXCEPT

    A. vision
    B. level of education
    C. hearing
    D. cognitive function

15. While recovering from surgery, a client avoids eye contact with the attending nurse, both while being cared for and when speaking. This is most likely a sign that the client is feeling

    A. ashamed
    B. fearful
    C. angry
    D. weak and defenseless

16. In nurse-client communication, which of the following variables is an emotional/psychological barrier to effective reception of a message?

    A. Using one's personal experience or frame of reference in interpreting
    B. Lack of context
    C. Distorting the message to comply with one's own expectations
    D. Insufficient vocabulary

17. Total parenteral nutrition (TPN) is usually contraindicated in clients whose gastrointestinal tracts are functional within _____ following an illness, surgery, or trauma.

    A. 24 hours
    B. 3 to 5 days
    C. 7 to 10 days
    D. 1 month

18. A client is undergoing oxygen therapy. The nurse can most effectively evaluate the effectiveness of this therapy by observing changes in

    A. blood volume
    B. serum electrolyte values
    C. arterial blood gases
    D. respiration

19. Which of the following nursing skills is most likely to be required during the pre-interaction phase of the nurse-client relationship?

    A. Analyzing one's one strengths and limitations
    B. Exploring relevant stressors
    C. Overcoming resistance behaviors
    D. Establishing trust

20. A nurse is instructed to give an IM injection into the ventrogluteal muscle. Each of the following would be a landmark used for this procedure, EXCEPT the

    A. lateral femoral condyle
    B. iliac crest
    C. greater trochanter
    D. anterior superior iliac spine

21. A nurse observes that a client's stool is green, loose, and has a strong odor. Based on this assessment, the next step of the nursing process that should be implemented is

    A. evaluating
    B. assessing
    C. implementing
    D. diagnosing

22. The main consequence of repeated vomiting is

    A. fluid and electrolyte loss
    B. dental caries
    C. metabolic alkalosis
    D. sleep disorder

23. Of the following medical conditions, which is most appropriate for the use of a nursing critical pathway?

    A. Knee replacement surgery
    B. Polyuria associated with pregnancy
    C. Viral infection acquired during travel
    D. Ear blockage by impacted cerumen

24. Coping or defense mechanisms that are used by clients include each of the following EXCEPT

    A. projection
    B. reinvention
    C. compensation
    D. denial

25. A client who recently suffered a herniated spinal disc complains of pain in her foot. During the nursing assessment, the nurse discovers no problems with the foot. The client's pain is best described as

    A. referred
    B. neuropathic
    C. phantom
    D. somatic

KEY (CORRECT ANSWERS)

1. B
2. B
3. B
4. A
5. A

6. C
7. A
8. C
9. A
10. A

11. A
12. A
13. A
14. B
15. D

16. C
17. C
18. C
19. A
20. A

21. D
22. A
23. A
24. B
25. A

EXAMINATION SECTION
TEST 1

DIRECTIONS: Each question or incomplete statement is followed by several suggested answers or completions. Select the one that BEST answers the question or completes the statement. *PRINT THE LETTER OF THE CORRECT ANSWER IN THE SPACE AT THE RIGHT.*

1. Which of the following is NOT a characteristic of the nursing care plan?

    A. It focuses on the present, rather than the future.
    B. It is based on identifiable health and nursing problems.
    C. It is a product of a deliberate systematic process.
    D. Its focus is holistic, rather than localized.

2. What method of wound debridement is generally least damaging?

    A. Scissors
    B. Chemical
    C. Wet to dry dressings
    D. Mechanical

3. Which of the following types of medications is LEAST likely to increase a client's risk of falling?

    A. antidepressants
    B. laxatives
    C. antibiotics
    D. diuretics

4. For most adults, healthy elimination patterns usually require a fluid intake of at least _____ ml daily.

    A. 750-1250
    B. 1500-2200
    C. 2000-3000
    D. 3500-5000

5. Which of the following is NOT a clinical guideline for assessing possible decubitus sites on a partially immobilized client?

    A. Avoiding incandescent light
    B. Inspecting for abrasions/excoriations
    C. Palpating skin temperature over pressure areas
    D. Elevating room temperature during assessment

6. During the assessment phase, a nurse will need to validate data when
    I. the data lack objectivity
    II. there is a discrepancy between what the client is saying and what the nurse is observing
    III. the data are not relevant to the client's presenting problem

    A. I only   B. I and II   C. II only   D. I, II and III

7. Following a mastectomy, a client says to a nurse: "The scar isn't as bad as I thought it was going to be." The client's eyes tear up and she looks anxious when she says this. Her message is an example of

    A. the Hawthorne effect
    B. congruence
    C. understatement
    D. metacommunication

8. In the _____ stage of the nursing process, the nurse ensures that the client is receiving the prescribed therapy at the appropriate times.

    A. evaluating
    B. diagnosing
    C. assessing
    D. planning/implementing

9. Among the following, the example that best represents "passive immunity" is

    A. a newborn receiving breast milk from his mother
    B. an infected person taking antibiotic medication
    C. an infected person producing antibodies
    D. a person receiving an influenza vaccine

10. The most common form of dementia is

    A. dementia due to Parkinson's disease
    B. AIDS dementia complex
    C. vascular dementia
    D. Alzheimer's disease

11. Which of the following positions puts the client at greatest risk for aspirating secretions?

    A. Sim's
    B. Fowler's
    C. Lateral
    D. Supine

12. The main factor that differentiates chronic pain from acute pain is that a client who is experiencing chronic pain is more likely to have

    A. a tissue injury
    B. a rapid pulse
    C. warm, dry skin
    D. dilated pupils

13. A client is refusing a blood transfusion because she says the procedure goes against her religious beliefs. The most appropriate action for the nurse to take is to

    A. notify a close family member who might persuade the client to undergo the procedure
    B. seek a court order compelling the client to submit to the procedure
    C. provide all the information the client needs to make an informed decision
    D. ask questions that probe the client's rationale, such as: "Do you think God would want for you to bleed to death?"

14. Which of the following nursing notes is an example of subjective data?

    A. Pulse is erratic
    B. Client's gait is unsteady
    C. Client's left hand is cool to the touch
    D. Client complains of headache

15. Each of the following would be an appropriate nursing intervention for a client with a chest drainage system, EXCEPT

    A. Placing the client in the Sim's position
    B. Monitoring the integrity of the drainage system
    C. Maintaining the water seal area of the unit
    D. Using clamps when appropriate

16. Which of the following is characteristic of the chronic cellular response phase of the inflammatory response?

    A. erythema
    B. hyperemia
    C. granuloma
    D. margination

17. When a nurse is preparing to teach a client, it is most useful for the nurse to know the client's

    A. educational background
    B. personal preferences
    C. family status
    D. developmental stage

18. For a client with sensory deficit, a nurse can appropriately increase environmental stimuli by

    A. using the television to provide intermittent auditory and visual stimuli
    B. installing a nightlight near the client's bed
    C. freeing the room of unnecessary clutter
    D. establishing a mealtime routine

19. A nurse informs a client: "Your arterial blood gases will be evaluated at seven p.m. tonight." Later, the client seems surprised and upset by the arterial blood draw. In informing the client about the procedure, the nurse's words probably required a greater measure of

    A. clarity
    B. simplicity
    C. timing
    D. tact

20. Which of the following is a term that denotes an isotonic gain of water and electrolytes? 20.____

    A. Dehydration
    B. Superhydration
    C. Fluid volume deficit
    D. Fluid volume excess

21. Of following clients, the one most likely to suffer a vitamin B deficiency would be the one who 21.____

    A. is on a low-residue diet
    B. abuses alcohol
    C. is pregnant
    D. does not regularly exercise

22. A nurse is attempting to establish a therapeutic environment for a confused elderly client. Of the following, the nurse should place the highest priority on 22.____

    A. a fixed routine
    B. supportive group interactions
    C. a trusting relationship
    D. a variety of activities

23. A client with a respiratory disease is only able to breathe when he is in an upright or standing position. In charting the client's condition, the nurse would use the medical term_____ to describe this condition. 23.____

    A. orthopnea
    B. tachypnea
    C. bradypnea
    D. apnea

24. A client is to have oxygen delivered in concentrations between 60 and 70 percent, at an average flow of 6.5 liters per minute. What type of mask should be used? 24.____

    A. Simple face mask
    B. Nonrebreather
    C. Partial rebreather
    D. Venturi

25. An elderly client was admitted to the emergency room three hours ago and has been hydrated with half-normal saline. During a subsequent assessment, the nurse observes a rapid pulse and shortness of breath. The nurse suspects that the client is showing signs of 25.____

    A. hypovolemia
    B. hypernatremia
    C. hypokalemia
    D. hypervolemia

KEY (CORRECT ANSWERS)

1. A
2. B
3. C
4. C
5. D

6. B
7. D
8. D
9. A
10. D

11. D
12. C
13. C
14. D
15. A

16. D
17. D
18. D
19. B
20. D

21. B
22. C
23. A
24. C
25. D

TEST 2

DIRECTIONS: Each question or incomplete statement is followed by several suggested answers or completions. Select the one that BEST answers the question or completes the statement. *PRINT THE LETTER OF THE CORRECT ANSWER IN THE SPACE AT THE RIGHT.*

1. In order to keep nurse-client communications therapeutic, the nurse should   1._____

    A. continue pushing the client toward some insights into his or her health behaviors
    B. make sure the conversation lasts for as long as the client wants to remain engaged
    C. make sure conversations remain goal-centered
    D. include prescriptive and directive language in the conversation

2. Which of the following body fluids is NOT associated with bloodborne pathogens?   2._____

    A. Vaginal secretions
    B. Pleural fluid
    C. Cerebrospinal fluid
    D. Nasal secretions

3. During an assessment interview, the nurse should use _____ questions to validate or clarify information.   3._____

    A. rhetorical
    B. direct
    C. open-ended
    D. reflective

4. A typical nursing intervention aimed at promoting the transport of oxygen and carbon dioxide is to   4._____

    A. reduce stress, in order to optimize cardiac output
    B. perform percussion, vibration, and postural drainage
    C. encourage coughing or deep breathing
    D. increase the amount of dietary fiber

5. A nurse is trying to help an elderly client regain urinary continence. Which of the following interventions would NOT be helpful?   5._____

    A. Teaching Kegel exercises
    B. Prompted voiding
    C. Restricting fluid intake
    D. Habit training/toilet scheduling

6. Kegel exercises are designed to strengthen the pubococcygeal muscle. Benefits associated with this exercise include   6._____
    I. reduced menstrual pain
    II. preparation for normal vaginal childbirth
    III. increased sexual gratification
    IV. improved urinary continence

    A. I and II   B. I, III and IV
    C. III and IV   D. I, II, III and IV

7. Each of the following is a risk factor that contributes to the formation of pressure ulcers, EXCEPT

    A. incontinence
    B. low blood protein
    C. inactivity
    D. lowered body temperature

8. Which of the following nursing activities poses the greatest risk for stress or injury to the nurse's back?

    A. Turning a client in bed
    B. Transferring a client in or out of bed
    C. Helping a client stand from a sitting position
    D. Helping a client walk

9. A nurse learns that a client does not appear to completely understand the risks of the surgery for which he is scheduled tomorrow. The nurse should notify the

    A. client's family
    B. surgical unit
    C. institution's administrative office
    D. surgeon

10. Client _____ behaviors are often encountered during the introductory phase of the nurse-client relationship, and may be due to difficulty in acknowledging the need for help, fear of exposing and facing feelings, and anxiety about changing behavior patterns.

    A. affiliative
    B. hostile
    C. resistive
    D. dependent

11. A nurse is establishing a therapeutic relationship with a client whose cultural background is vastly different from his own. It is important for the nurse, in establishing this relationship, to

    A. not mention the difference to the client, but remain aware of it throughout interactions
    B. ignore or minimize the difference
    C. wait for the client to mention the difference
    D. acknowledge the difference forthrightly

12. Together, the nurse and client devise a nursing care plan that includes the goal of maintaining fluid and electrolyte balances within normal limits. Each of the following would be an evaluation that could help measure outcomes for this goal, EXCEPT

    A. monitoring bowel elimination patterns
    B. weighing the client
    C. palpation for edema and skin breakdown
    D. monitoring vital signs for tachycardia, dysrhythmias, hypertension, and dyspnea

13. Under the nurse's teaching, a client is learning how to use crutches after a knee operation. The nurse should instruct the client to do each of the following, EXCEPT to

    A. adjust the length of the crutches frequently and independently, until they are comfortable
    B. regularly inspect the crutch tips
    C. remain as erect as possible when using them
    D. use the arms, and not the armpit pads, to support weight

14. A nurse is teaching a 24-year-old client with insulin-dependent diabetes to manage his diet, sugars, and insulin regimen. The client will most likely be interested in learning this information from the nurse if the nurse

    A. makes the client sufficiently aware that the disease can be life-threatening
    B. reminds the client that he has several family members who rely on him to remain healthy and able-bodied
    C. is able to fully communicate the future implications of uncontrolled diabetes
    D. is able to relate the need for control of certain factors in the client's present-day life

15. A client reports to the emergency department complaining of angina and shortness of breath. Before performing a physical assessment of this client, the nurse obtains a history. Which of the following data will be relevant for this client?

    A. History of diabetes or smoking
    B. History of atrial fibrillation
    C. History of taking dietary supplements
    D. Allergy history

16. Dorothea Orem's nursing model is based on the principle that

    A. the best people to care for a client are his or her family, with help from medical professionals
    B. all clients wish to care for themselves
    C. the nurse acts as a gatekeeper, both for information and therapeutic care
    D. the client is an interrelated set of systems: biological, psychological, and social

17. A nurse who is preparing a client for a sigmoidoscopy would

    A. explain to the client that she will have to swallow a chalky substance before the examination
    B. explain the client that no fluids can be ingested within 24 hours prior to the examination
    C. administer an enema on the morning of the examination
    D. collect a stool specimen from the client

18. A nurse is preparing a client for a series of diagnostic tests. When explaining the tests to the client, the nurse should

    A. provide specific and detailed information about each test involved in the series
    B. provide minimal answers to client questions if the client appears anxious
    C. provide enough information to help the client understand the procedures, but not so much as to overwhelm her
    D. wait until just prior to each test, in order to postpone unnecessary anxiety

19. The leading cause of injury in older adults is

    A. medication dosage error
    B. automobile accidents
    C. exposure/hypothermia
    D. falling

20. A client has end stage renal disease. Upon reporting for his shift, the nurse learns that the client's vital signs have been dropping throughout the day. The nurse enters the client's room and sees that her dentures and bed linens are dirty, and her hair is unkempt. His plan for intervention should include

    A. recommending that the client remove her dentures
    B. asking the client what she needs to be more comfortable
    C. telling the client that her hair must be washed
    D. asking the client if she can get herself out of bed so that the linens can be changed

21. The nurse who wants to assess a client's temperature at its highest daily level should take temperature readings at

    A. 8 p.m. and midnight
    B. 3 p.m. and 9 p.m.
    C. noon and 5 p.m.
    D. 3 a.m. and 7 a.m.

22. A client has been placed on a soft diet. Which of the following foods would NOT be allowed?

    A. Tofu
    B. Oatmeal
    C. Raisins
    D. Yogurt

23. A client's medication order reads "Keflex 250 mg po." The drug is available as Keflex 125 mg/ml. The nurse should give _____ ml.

    A. 2
    B. 12
    C. 20
    D. 45

24. A nurse who, throughout every facet of his work, shows that he is answerable to himself and those in authority is demonstrating that he is

    A. accountable
    B. responsible
    C. ethical
    D. beneficent

25. A nurse finds a client's distraught mother in the client's room, long after visiting hours have been ended. The client is asleep. The nurse tells the mother in a calm, patient voice that she will have to go home for the night. The mother responds, but the nurse does not attend to her response because he is thinking that the institution's policy, in this case, is not helpful to the client or his family. This kind of distraction in communication is known as

   A. scapegoating
   B. intrapersonal communication
   C. derailing
   D. cross-talk

KEY (CORRECT ANSWERS)

1.	C	11.	D
2.	D	12.	A
3.	B	13.	A
4.	A	14.	D
5.	C	15.	A
6.	C	16.	B
7.	D	17.	C
8.	B	18.	C
9.	D	19.	D
10.	C	20.	B
21.	A		
22.	C		
23.	A		
24.	A		
25.	B		

TEST 3

DIRECTIONS: Each question or incomplete statement is followed by several suggested answers or completions. Select the one that BEST answers the question or completes the statement. *PRINT THE LETTER OF THE CORRECT ANSWER IN THE SPACE AT THE RIGHT.*

1. A therapeutic relationship
    I. involves an emotional commitment
    II. is goal-directed
    III. is planned
    IV. focuses on client needs

    A. I and II
    B. I, II and III
    C. II, III and IV
    D. I, II, III and IV

    1.____

2. A brachial pulse is taken typically to

    A. obtain the most accurate reading possible
    B. measure blood pressure
    C. to calculate resting heart rate
    D. determine cerebral circulation

    2.____

3. The most important difference between a nursing diagnosis and a medical diagnosis is that

    A. medical diagnoses are evidence-based, while nursing diagnoses are anecdotal
    B. nurses are not allowed to engage in medical diagnosis
    C. nursing diagnoses focus on human responses to stimuli, while medical diagnoses focus on the disease process.
    D. nursing diagnoses focus on health promotion, while medical diagnoses focus on treatment

    3.____

4. A client's wound is draining thick yellow material. Which of the following descriptions would be LEAST appropriate in describing the wound?

    A. Purulent
    B. Pyogenic
    C. Serous
    D. Suppurative

    4.____

5. A client has been admitted to the emergency room complaining of a headache and weakness. The nurse observes that she appears confused and has warm, flushed skin. Her vital signs are as follows: T 101.8; HR 124; R 22; and BP 128/90. A blood gas sample was taken on room air, with the following results: pH 7.35; pCO_2 58; pO_2 70; HCO_3 23. The client is at risk for

    A. metabolic acidosis
    B. metabolic alkalosis
    C. respiratory acidosis
    D. respiratory alkalosis

    5.____

6. A client is referred to a nurse by a local women's shelter, where she has fled a violent marriage. The client tells the nurse she is having trouble deciding whether to continue the relationship with her husband. The most appropriate nursing diagnosis for this client is

   A. risk for injury
   B. readiness for enhanced spiritual well-being
   C. decisional conflict
   D. energy field disturbance

7. Which of the following is LEAST likely to be a site for a skinfold test during a nursing assessment?

   A. Subiliac
   B. Triceps
   C. Subscapula
   D. Thigh

8. Weight loss, described as "severe" once it exceeds _____ percent, is one of the clinical signs of fluid volume deficit.

   A. 5
   B. 8
   C. 12
   D. 20

9. Which of the following is NOT a fluid/electrolyte condition that is typically caused by stress?

   A. Hypervolemia
   B. Reduced cellular metabolism
   C. Sodium retention
   D. Water retention

10. When evaluating a family's coping resources, a nurse should consider the

    A. structure of the family
    B. availability of support
    C. individual roles of family members
    D. family's preventive health practices

11. Which of the following is MOST likely to be a therapeutic communication technique when used by a nurse?

    A. Challenging
    B. Advising
    C. Disagreeing
    D. Restating

12. A client who has recently broken his arm complains of a dull, generalized pain along his forearm. This type of pain is best described as

    A. somatic   B. cutaneous
    C. phantom   D. visceral

13. A nurse is teaching a client about a low-cholesterol diet. Which of the following activities is MOST likely to facilitate retention?

    A. breaking down the lesson into individual units that are followed by quizzes
    B. under the nurse's supervision, having the client develop a weekly menu by selecting foods
    C. assigning reading and computer-aided activities
    D. using visual aids with bold line drawings

13.____

14. Which of the following nursing interventions is MOST appropriate for a client with a urinary tract infection?

    A. Facilitate access to toilet
    B. Encourage fluid intake
    C. Decrease calcium intake
    D. Teach Kegel exercises

14.____

15. With a completely or partially immobilized client, many nursing interventions for the respiratory system are aimed at promoting expansion of the chest and lungs. Of the following, the most effective intervention for this purpose is

    A. isometric exercises
    B. physiotherapy
    C. frequent position changes
    D. aerobic exercise

15.____

16. Together, a nurse and client are working on a plan to reduce the client's health risk factors. Which of the following interventions would be LEAST effective in assisting the client?

    A. Asking the client identify three goals for change
    B. Helping the client compose a plan for change
    C. Allowing the client to establish a reasonable time period for change
    D. Writing up a behavioral plan and then asking the client to adhere to it

16.____

17. The open systems model of nursing care is driven by the principle that communication should be used by the nurse to

    A. promote wellness
    B. heal the client
    C. widen the client's support network
    D. help the client adapt to his or her environment

17.____

18. The most appropriate demonstration of critical thinking by an inexperienced nurse would occur when he

    A. asks the client many focused questions
    B. relies on what he has witnessed other nurses do in similar situations
    C. admits uncertainty about how to perform a procedure, and asking for help
    D. studies the institutional policies and procedures manual

18.____

19. A client is to undergo a test for occult blood in the stool. For three days prior to the test, it is important for the client to take each of the following precautions, EXCEPT to

    A. avoid oral iron supplements
    B. avoid alcohol or caffeine
    C. undergo an assessment for hemorrhoids
    D. avoid the ingestion of red meat

20. Which of the following processes in nursing diagnosis occurs FIRST?

    A. Making a decision on the problem based on validation
    B. Observing/noting changes in physical status
    C. Taking necessary steps to rule out other hypotheses
    D. Determining the possible alternatives that could have caused changes in physical status

21. A client will most likely respond favorably to a nurse's verbal communication if the nurse

    A. remains professional and uses medical and technical terms for conditions and procedures
    B. opens up and reveals something about himself during communication
    C. maintains the same tone of voice throughout the conversation
    D. uses consistency in both verbal and nonverbal communication

22. Serum osmolality values are used during the assessment of a client's fluid and electrolyte balance, primarily to measure the extent of

    A. hypervolemia
    B. fluid volume excess
    C. dehydration
    D. fluid volume deficit

23. Before reminding a client of the importance of consistently taking his prescribed medication on schedule, a nurse decides what tone of voice to use and what gestures, if any, will be used to reinforce the message. The nurse is engaging in a process known as

    A. verbal cues
    B. inductive bias
    C. sending
    D. encoding

24. "To Err is Human: Building a Safer Health System," the influential report published by the Institute of Medicine in 2000, between 44,000 and 98,000 people die in the United States each year from _____ more than die from motor vehicle accidents, breast cancer, or Alzheimer's disease.

    A. heart disease
    B. illegal drug use
    C. AIDS
    D. medical errors

25. A nurse is administering oxygen to a client with emphysema. The nurse uses an oxygen analyzer to monitor levels of oxygen, knowing that high levels of oxygen over long periods of time are most likely to cause   25._____

   A. hyperventilation
   B. damage to the retina and cornea
   C. irreversible brain damage
   D. pulmonary edema

KEY (CORRECT ANSWERS)

1. C	11. D
2. B	12. A
3. C	13. B
4. C	14. B
5. C	15. C
6. C	16. D
7. A	17. D
8. B	18. C
9. B	19. B
10. B	20. B

21. D
22. C
23. D
24. D
25. B

EXAMINATION SECTION
TEST 1

DIRECTIONS: Each question or incomplete statement is followed by several suggested answers or completions. Select the one that BEST answers the question or completes the statement. *PRINT THE LETTER OF THE CORRECT ANSWER IN THE SPACE AT THE RIGHT.*

1. The nurse-client relationship is characterized by each of the following, EXCEPT   1.____

    A. positive regard
    B. therapeutic self-disclosure
    C. abstraction
    D. empathy

2. Which of the following is an example of an open-ended question?   2.____

    A. Did you leave the bed to urinate last night?
    B. When did you first begin to notice the pain?
    C. Is somebody coming to pick you up this morning?
    D. What happened to your shoulder?

3. Of the following, which is LEAST likely to cause REM sleep deprivation?   3.____

    A. A regularly scheduled 60-hour work week
    B. Sleep apnea
    C. Barbiturates
    D. Alcohol

4. When assessing a client's communication abilities, a nurse needs to evaluate both the client's communication style and   4.____

    A. impairments or barriers to communication
    B. education level
    C. medical history
    D. posture

5. The term "aphagia" refers to   5.____

    A. the inability to swallow
    B. the inability to speak
    C. difficult or painful swallowing
    D. an absence of white blood cells

6. During the assessment phase, a nurse acquires each of the following items of data. Which would require validation?   6.____

    A. The client says she feels feverish
    B. The client's pulse is 102
    C. The client's blood pressure is 112/65
    D. The client's chart indicates a history of asthma

7. During the assessment interview, a nurse attempts to use active listening skills. Which of the following is an element of this skill set?

   A. Responding quickly to the client and trying to summarize the client's statements
   B. Interrupting the client only when clarification is needed
   C. Asking for crucial items of information
   D. Listening for principal themes in the client's communication

8. Each of the following is a recognized stage in the body's inflammatory response to infection, EXCEPT

   A. exudate
   B. vascular response
   C. passive immunity
   D. reparation

9. Generally, a humidifying device will be required when oxygen is administered to a client at a flow rate of _____ liters/minute or more.

   A. 2
   B. 4
   C. 6
   D. 8

10. During an assessment interview, a nurse attempts to assess the client's personal identity. Which of the following questions is an appropriate means of assessing this?

    A. What kind of people do you most enjoy being around?
    B. Do you have any meaningful relationships with family members?
    C. Do you think this problem has anything to do with your choices or behaviors?
    D. If you could change anything about yourself, what would it be?

11. Possible causes of polyuria include each of the following, EXCEPT

    A. extremely low fluid intake
    B. congestive heart failure
    C. intestinal obstruction
    D. liver failure

12. In nursing, a process recording is primarily useful for

    A. insuring that all interventions and medications are having the desired effects
    B. ensuring that the nurse adheres to an established care plan
    C. analyzing the effectiveness of nurse-client communication in modifying client behaviors
    D. establishing a therapeutic relationship

13. When a client develops contracts the human immunodeficiency virus (HIV), he loses _____ immunity.

    A. passive
    B. adaptive
    C. cellular
    D. humoral

14. A client with non-Hodgkin's lymphoma is receiving leurocristine. The nurse should make sure the client's diet is

    A. low-fat
    B. high in fluids but low in residue
    C. low in protein, but with increased iron
    D. high in fluids and dietary fiber

15. A client's medication order reads "Chlorpropamide 250 mg qd. The medication is available as Diabinese, .25 gram tablets. How many tablets should the nurse give to the client in one dose?

    A. half
    B. 1
    C. one-and-half
    D. 2

16. A sleep history taken during a nursing assessment typically includes each of the following, EXCEPT

    A. content of dreams
    B. bedtime rituals
    C. use of sleep medications
    D. client satisfaction with sleep

17. A 38-year-old client is admitted to the hospital with a diagnosis of chronic renal insufficiency. He is weak, hypotensive, and has low sodium and high potassium levels. The focus of his nursing care plan should be

    A. restoring electrolyte balance
    B. increasing urinary output
    C. increasing carbohydrate intake
    D. postural drainage

18. A client visits a clinic with a twisted ankle that has swollen. Of the following chronic conditions, which would contraindicate the use of ice on the ankle?

    A. Chronic obstructive pulmonary disease
    B. Osteoporosis
    C. Glaucoma
    D. Diabetes mellitus

19. Prior to a surgical procedure, a client asks the nurse to stay and pray with him and his wife. The nurse is an agnostic who does not attend church services and has never prayed before. The most appropriate nursing action would for the nurse to

    A. stay with the client and either join in the prayer or remain silent
    B. explain that prayer is not a part of her personal belief system
    C. try to explain with humor that she is an agnostic and her prayers are unlikely to do any good
    D. offer to have the hospital chaplain perform a service

20. Which of the following nursing interventions is LEAST appropriate for a client with chronic renal failure?

    A. Hourly assessment for hyper- or hypovolemia
    B. Promote maintenance of skin integrity
    C. Hourly assessment for signs of uremia
    D. Monitor and prevent changes in fluid and electrolyte balance

21. During auscultation, the nurse notes a high-pitched musical sound during expiration. This would be documented as

    A. rhonchi
    B. rales
    C. crepitations
    D. wheeze

22. Each of the following is involved in a typical nutritional assessment, EXCEPT

    A. the dietary history
    B. a comparison of weight to body build
    C. mid-upper arm circumference measurement
    D. girth measurements

23. Which of the following nursing diagnoses is written in PES format?

    A. Potential for impaired skin integrity related to immobility
    B. Impaired communication related to laryngectomy, as manifested by an inability to talk,
    C. At risk for aspiration
    D. Decreased caloric intake related to altered nutrition: Less than body requirements

24. A nurse is administering oxygen to a client with emphysema. An oxygen analyzer is used to monitor levels of oxygen, and is calibrated using room air, which is about _____ percent oxygen

    A. 10
    B. 20
    C. 40
    D. 60

25. A father is frustrated because his five-year-old son cannot stay dry at night. The most appropriate suggestion by the nurse would be that

    A. bedwetting is often a sign of an underlying psychological problem
    B. the father should ask the doctor about the possibility of prescribing Desmopressin
    C. while frustrating, bedwetting is a condition that is not normally appropriate for treatment until a child reaches the age of six or seven
    D. the child should be awakened at the same time every night to void his bladder

KEY (CORRECT ANSWERS)

1.	C	11.	A
2.	D	12.	C
3.	A	13.	C
4.	A	14.	D
5.	A	15.	B
6.	A	16.	A
7.	D	17.	A
8.	C	18.	D
9.	A	19.	A
10.	D	20.	A

21. D
22. D
23. B
24. B
25. C

TEST 2

DIRECTIONS: Each question or incomplete statement is followed by several suggested answers or completions. Select the one that BEST answers the question or completes the statement. *PRINT THE LETTER OF THE CORRECT ANSWER IN THE SPACE AT THE RIGHT.*

1. In planning a menu for a vegetarian client, the nurse will need to take special care that the client's food contains adequate amounts of

    A. protein
    B. carbohydrate
    C. fiber
    D. vitamin A

2. The word "macule" refers to a

    A. flat area of discoloration on the skin
    B. raised or elevated area
    C. blister-like raised area filled with fluid
    D. raised area containing pus

3. Which of the following is MOST likely to be the causative factor in ischemia?

    A. aneurysm
    B. respiratory distress
    C. atherosclerosis
    D. anemia

4. During the assessment phase of the nursing process, the nurse applies critical thinking when she

    A. thinks ahead to the therapeutic goals that are likely to be established
    B. asks closed-ended questions
    C. expresses doubt about the data provided by the client
    D. asks questions that are culturally sensitive

5. The most common infecting organism associated with nosocomial infections is

    A. Enterococcus
    B. Staphylococcus aureus
    C. Lactobacillus
    D. E. coli

6. In the following nursing diagnosis-Ineffective airway clearance related to decreased energy as manifested by an ineffective cough-the etiology of the diagnosis is represented by

    A. decreased energy
    B. an ineffective cough
    C. as manifested by
    D. ineffective airway clearance

7. A client with gastroenteritis and severe diarrhea is MOST at risk for losing excessive amounts of

    A. chloride
    B. potassium
    C. sodium
    D. phosphate

8. Which of the following behaviors-on the part of the nurse-is known to inhibit effective nurse-client communication?

    A. Maintaining silence
    B. Stating observations
    C. Paraphrasing
    D. Showing approval or disapproval

9. Typically, a nurse may facilitate pulmonary ventilation through each of the following means, EXCEPT

    A. suctioning
    B. stress reduction
    C. percussion
    D. hydration

10. Of the following, which as at greatest risk for developing an upper respiratory infection?

    A. 30-year-old with Stage I HIV infection
    B. 45-year-old pregnant client
    C. 60-year-old nonsmoker
    D. 4-year-old preschooler

11. While bathing a client, the nurse assesses the client's skin. Which of the following would necessitate a referral to another health professional?

    A. Pitted edema at the ankles
    B. Rough, flaking skin in exposed areas
    C. Keratosis pilaris
    D. Angular stomatitis

12. A client with hyperpnea

    A. is hyperventilating
    B. will need to exercise or otherwise raise his heart rate to improve blood oxygenation
    C. is experiencing an excessively high rate of alveolar ventilation
    D. presents a prolonged gasping inspiration followed by a very short, usually inefficient, expiration

13. A client with obesity is at greater risk of suffering _____ postoperatively than a client who is not obese.

    A. infection
    B. respiratory distress
    C. anaphylaxis
    D. delayed healing

14. A client has not adhered to a diet designed to manage her diabetes. Of the following, which statement or question by the nurse would be MOST likely to motivate the client to comply with dietary restrictions?

    A. I understand the diet is hard for you to stick to. Can you tell me why you find it so difficult?
    B. I'm having trouble understanding why you won't stick to the diet when we agreed upon it together.
    C. The diet has been designed to lengthen your life expectancy. Do you understand the consequences if you don't adhere to it?
    D. Is there somebody at home who can make sure you adhere to the diet?

15. Which of the following is an interdependent nursing action?

    A. Developing a nursing care plan
    B. Preparing a client for diagnostic tests
    C. Changing sterile dressings
    D. Teaching a client about hygiene

16. Which of the following communication tasks is typically part of the planning phase of the nursing process?

    A. Seeking the involvement of additional health resources
    B. Discussing methods of implementation with client
    C. Meeting the client
    D. Examining the need for adjustments and changes

17. For a client with mild hypothermia, the most appropriate intervention is

    A. administering warm IV fluids
    B. applying blankets
    C. applying an electric blanket
    D. turning up the room thermostat

18. Which of the following is NOT a therapeutic communication technique?

    A. Stating observations
    B. Clarifying
    C. Summarizing
    D. Offering opinions

19. During the psychosocial assessment of an 8-year-old client, it would be most helpful for the nurse to

    A. read the client a story or play a video prior to the interview
    B. provide some toys for the client to play with during the interview
    C. provide a nutritious snack
    D. establish a quiet and private setting

20. A nurse who wants a client to obtain maximum benefits after postural drainage should encourage the client to

    A. use bronchodilators
    B. remain lying down

C. elevate the feet
D. cough deeply

21. A nurse is developing a nutrition program for 6- and 7-year-old children. Given known health problems for children in this age group, the program should include

    A. distinguishing between HDL and LDL cholesterol
    B. identifying foods that contain water-soluble vitamins
    C. recognizing the importance of taking daily vitamin supplements
    D. identifying foods that may contribute to obesity

21.____

22. The most likely reaction of a client who has been recently transferred to the intensive care unit would be

    A. defiance
    B. confusion
    C. fear
    D. relief

22.____

23. When assessing a client's pain, the most important factor to consider is the

    A. likelihood that the pain will interfere with normal functioning
    B. client's own perception of the pain
    C. client's vital signs
    D. underlying cause of the pain

23.____

24. During the orientation stage of an initial interview with the client, the nurse should

    A. establish his authority and background in interviewing clients
    B. indicate what client health behaviors will be most desirable
    C. stick to closed questioning
    D. explain the purpose of the interview

24.____

25. A doctor has prescribed 5 tablespoons of an anti-diarrhea medication. The nurse's equipment is only marked for metric measurements. How many ml will the nurse administer?

    A. 12
    B. 32.5
    C. 75
    D. 130

25.____

KEY (CORRECT ANSWERS)

1. A
2. A
3. C
4. D
5. D

6. A
7. B
8. D
9. B
10. D

11. A
12. C
13. D
14. A
15. A

16. B
17. B
18. D
19. D
20. D

21. D
22. C
23. B
24. D
25. C

TEST 3

DIRECTIONS: Each question or incomplete statement is followed by several suggested answers or completions. Select the one that BEST answers the question or completes the statement. *PRINT THE LETTER OF THE CORRECT ANSWER IN THE SPACE AT THE RIGHT.*

1. Nontherapeutic responses to client concerns include

    A. Reflecting
    B. Focusing
    C. Summarizing
    D. Probing

1.____

2. A nurse is working with a client who needs to learn how to perform her own colostomy care. It is most important that the nurse assess and facilitate

    A. readiness
    B. comfort
    C. motivation
    D. knowledge

2.____

3. The early treatment of diabetic acidosis would involve

    A. NPH insulin
    B. Respiratory intubation
    C. IV fluids
    D. Restricted sodium intake

3.____

4. Which of the following nursing skills is MOST likely to be required during the termination phase of the nurse-client relationship?

    A. Summarizing
    B. Clarifying
    C. Goal-setting
    D. Risk-taking

4.____

5. For a client who has a significant body odor, the most appropriate solution is

    A. a lesson in personal hygiene
    B. a bath or shower
    C. an alcohol-based deodorant
    D. antiperspirant

5.____

6. Symptoms of alveolar hyperventilation include

    A. numbness
    B. warm, dry skin
    C. pallor
    D. convulsions

6.____

155

7. The nurse is preparing to communicate discharge information to an elderly client of Chinese descent who speaks English well, but it is his second language. The best way to communicate with this client is to

    A. provide brief, simple explanations, and speak slowly
    B. provide some literature that he can read on his own later
    C. find an interpreter or family member to help
    D. provide comprehensive explanations of all information

8. Which phase of the nursing process involves the systematic and continuous collection, organization, validation, and documentation of data?

    A. Evaluating
    B. Assessing
    C. Planning
    D. Diagnosing

9. During the nursing assessment of a client with heart disease, the nurse becomes concerned that the client might be suffering from hypoxia. Each of the following is a clinical sign of hypoxia, EXCEPT

    A. intercostal retraction
    B. deep, rapid breaths
    C. cyanosis
    D. flaring nostrils

10. Digitalis preparations often involve the depletion of _____ as a side effect.

    A. phosphate
    B. potassium
    C. iron
    D. calcium

11. The label on a bottle of atropine states that the strength of each tablet is "gr 1/120." The client's medication order says that she should receive 0.5 g of atropine. The nurse should give the client _____ tablet.

    A. half
    B. 1
    C. one-and-half
    D. 2

12. A client complains of polyuria, pain on urination, and an unpleasant smell. The nurse calls for a urine sample. Which of the following is the most likely problem?

    A. Renal calculi
    B. Urinary tract infection
    C. Glomerulonephritis
    D. Acute renal failure

13. _____ infections are defined as those due to any aspect of medical therapy.

    A. Occult
    B. Nosocomial

C. Iatrogenic
D. Exanthematic

14. When ending an interview, the most appropriate communication technique for the nurse to use is usually

    A. a firm handshake
    B. reflecting
    C. summarizing
    D. self-disclosure

15. A 13-year-old client is experiencing painful abdominal cramps during menstruation. The most appropriate intervention for this would be to instruct the client to

    A. perform mild stretching exercises of the lower back and abdominal muscles
    B. rest and apply an ice pack to the abdomen
    C. decrease fluid intake
    D. rest and apply warmth to the abdomen

16. A nurse is developing an initial plan of care for a client. The plan should include

    A. a request for possible psychological consultation
    B. the client's vital signs on admission
    C. a nursing diagnosis
    D. a list of medications currently taken by the client

17. A client is about to undergo an adrenalectomy. It is MOST important for the nurse to insure _____ during the preoperative period.

    A. adequate nutrition
    B. increased fluid intake
    C. complete rest
    D. electrolyte balance

18. Which of the following clients might be legally allowed to give informed consent to a medical procedure?

    A. A client who is under sedation
    B. A client who experiences intermittent episodes of dementia who appears lucid at the time of consent
    C. An unconscious client
    D. A client whose injury or disability does not enable her to sign the consent form

19. A client who has recently suffered a laceration to her forehead complains of a throbbing localized pain on the surface of her head. This type of pain is best described as

    A. somatic
    B. neuropathic
    C. cutaneous
    D. visceral

20. A nursing care plan includes the goal of appropriate client response to stimuli. Which of the following outcomes would MOST clearly show that this goal has been met?

    A. Client is able to formulate sounds within 24 hours of admission
    B. Client and family openly discuss plans for discharge with a social worker by the fifth day of hospitalization
    C. Client is able to transmit a clear message to a nurse or family member by the second day of hospitalization
    D. Client is able to nonverbally acknowledge the receipt of a verbal message within 24 hours of admission

21. To examine the size of a client's liver, the nurse moves her hands over the surface of the client's abdomen. This examination technique is known as

    A. auscultation
    B. percussion
    C. palpation
    D. inspection

22. In communicating with toddlers or preschoolers, a nurse should be sure to

    A. prevent the child from handling equipment
    B. avoid nonverbal cues
    C. deflect difficult questions by offering a toy or snack
    D. focus the conversation on the child's personal needs and concerns

23. Which of the following is an example of ablative surgery?

    A. Mitral valve replacement
    B. Colostomy
    C. Tonsillectomy
    D. Arthroplasty

24. Likely causes of fluid volume deficit include each of the following, EXCEPT

    A. excess steroid intake
    B. bleeding
    C. third-space movement
    D. decreased fluid intake

25. A client has been placed on a low-residue diet. Which of the following foods would NOT be allowed?

    A. Oatmeal
    B. Butter
    C. Cottage Cheese
    D. Canned, peeled vegetables

KEY (CORRECT ANSWERS)

1.	D	11.	B
2.	A	12.	B
3.	C	13.	C
4.	A	14.	C
5.	B	15.	D
6.	A	16.	C
7.	A	17.	C
8.	B	18.	D
9.	B	19.	C
10.	B	20.	D

21. C
22. D
23. C
24. A
25. A

BASIC NURSING PROCEDURES: FUNDAMENTAL NURSING CARE OF THE PATIENT

TABLE OF CONTENTS

		Page
1.	Morning Care	1
2.	Oral Hygiene	2
3.	Special Mouth Care	3
4.	Care of Dentures	5
5.	Bed Bath	6
6.	Making an Unoccupied Bed	8
7.	Making an Occupied Bed	12
8.	Serving Diets from Food Cart	16
9.	Central Tray Service	18
10.	Care of Ice Machine and Handling of Ice, Bedside Pitchers and Glasses	19
11.	Feeding the Helpless Patient	21
12.	Evening Care	22
13.	Care of the Seriously Ill Patient	23

BASIC NURSING PROCEDURES: FUNDAMENTAL NURSING CARE OF THE PATIENT

1. MORNING CARE

PURPOSE

To refresh and prepare patient for breakfast.

EQUIPMENT

Basin of warm water
Towel, washcloth and soap
Toothbrush and dentifrice/mouthwash
Curved basin
Glass of water
Comb

PROCEDURE

1. Clear bedside stand or overbed table for food tray.
2. Offer bedpan and urinal.
3. Wash patient's face and hands.
4. Give oral hygiene.
5. Place patient in a comfortable position for breakfast.
6. Comb hair.

POINTS TO EMPHASIZE

1. Morning care is given before breakfast by night corpsman.
2. Assist handicapped, aged or patients on complete bed rest.

CARE OF EQUIPMENT

Wash, dry and replace equipment.

2. ORAL HYGIENE

PURPOSE

To keep mouth clean.
To refresh patient.
To prevent infection and complications in the oral cavity.
To stimulate appetite.

EQUIPMENT

Glass of water
Curved basin
Toothbrush and dentifrice - electric toothbrush if available
Mouth wash
Towel
Drinking tubes as necessary

PROCEDURE

1. A patient who is able to help himself:
    a. Place patient in comfortable position.
    b. Arrange equipment on bedside table within his reach.

2. A patient who needs assistance:
    a. Place patient in comfortable position.
    b. Place towel under his chin and over bedding.
    c. Moisten brush, apply dentifrice and hand to the patient.
    d. Hold curved basin under his chin while he cleanses his teeth and mouth.
    e. Remove basin. Wipe lips and chin with towel.

POINTS TO EMPHASIZE

Oral hygiene is particularly important for patients
    a. who are not taking food and fluid by mouth
    b. with nasogastric tubes
    c. with productive coughs
    d. who are receiving oxygen therapy

CARE OF EQUIPMENT

Wash equipment with soap and hot water, rinse, dry and put away.

3. SPECIAL MOUTH CARE

PURPOSE

To cleanse and refresh mouth.
To prevent infection.

EQUIPMENT

Electric toothbrush if available
Tray with:
- Mineral oil or cold cream
- Lemon-glycerine applicators
- Paper bag
- Drinking tubes or straws
- Applicators and gauze sponges
- Curved basin
- Paper wipes
- Bulb syringe

Cleansing agents

- Tooth paste
- Equal parts of hydrogen peroxide and water
- Mouthwash

Glass of water
Suction machine for unconscious patient

PROCEDURE

1. Tell patient what you are going to do.
2. Turn patient's head to one side.
3. Brush teeth and gums.
4. When it is not possible to brush teeth and gums, moisten applicator with a cleansing agent and use for cleaning oral cavity and teeth.
5. Assist patient to rinse mouth with water.
6. If patient is unable to use drinking tube, gently irrigate the mouth with a syringe directing the flow of water to side of mouth.
7. Apply lubricant to lips.

For Unconscious Patient

Use suction machine.

SPECIAL MOUTH CARE (Continued)

POINTS TO EMPHASIZE
1. Extreme care should be exercised to prevent injury to the gums.
2. Position patient carefully to prevent aspiration of fluids.
3. Caution patient not to swallow mouthwash.

CARE OF EQUIPMENT

Dispose of applicator and soiled gauze. Clean equipment and restock tray.

4. CARE OF DENTURES

PURPOSE

To aid in keeping mouth in good condition.
To cleanse the teeth.

EQUIPMENT

Container for dentures
Toothbrush and dentifrice
Glass of water
Mouthwash
Curved basin
Towel
Paper towels

PROCEDURE

1. Have patient rinse mouth with mouthwash.
2. Remove dentures. Place them in container.
3. Have patient brush tongue and gums with mouth-wash.
4. Place a basin under tap in sink and place paper towels in basin. Fill basin with cold water.
5. Hold dentures over basin and under cold running water. Wash with brush and dentifrice.
6. Place dentures in container of cold water. Take to patient's bedside.
7. Replace wet dentures.

POINTS TO EMPHASIZE

1. Handle dentures carefully to prevent breakage.
2. When not in use, dentures should be placed in covered container of cold water and placed in top drawer of locker.
3. Give special attention to the inner surfaces of clips used to hold bridge work or partial plates in place.

CARE OF EQUIPMENT

Wash equipment, rinse, dry and put away.

5. BED BATH

PURPOSE

To cleanse the skin.
To stimulate the circulation.
To observe the patient mentally and physically.
To aid in elimination.

EQUIPMENT

Linen and pajamas as required
Half filled basin of water
Bar of soap
Rubbing alcohol/skin lotion
Bedpan and urinal with cover
Bed screens

PROCEDURE

1. Tell patient what you are going to do.
2. Screen patient.
3. Offer bedpan and urinal.
4. Shave patient or allow patient to shave himself.
5. Lower backrest and knee rest if physical condition permits.
6. Loosen top bedding at foot and sides of bed.
7. Remove pillow and place on chair.
8. Remove and fold bedspread and blanket. Place on back of chair.
9. Remove pajamas and place on chair.
10. Assist patient to near side of bed.
11. Bathe the patient:

    a. Eyes:
        (1) Do not use soap.
        (2) Clean from inner to outer corner of eye.

    b. Face, neck and ears.
    c. Far arm.
    d. Place hand in basin and clean nails.
    e. Near arm.
    f. Place hand in basin and clean nails.
    g. Chest.
    h. Abdomen.

BED BATH (Continued)

PROCEDURE (Continued)

12.
- i. Far leg, foot and nails. Place foot in basin when possible.
- j. Near leg, foot and nails. Place foot in basin when possible.
- k. Change water. l. Back and buttocks.
- m. Genitals and rectal area.

13. Give back rub.
14. Put on pajamas.
15. Comb hair.
16. Make bed.
17. Adjust bed to patient's comfort unless contrain-dicated.

POINTS TO EMPHASIZE

1. Give bed baths daily and P.R.N.
2. Give oral hygiene before bath.
3. Avoid drafts which might cause chilling.
4. Use bath towel under all parts to aid in keeping the bed linen as dry as possible.
5. Change bath water after washing lower extremities and as necessary.
6. Be sure all soap film is rinsed from body to prevent skin irritation.
7. Keep patient well draped at all times.
8. Observe and chart the condition of the skin in regard to lesions, rashes and reddened areas.
9. Pillow should be removed unless contraindicated to give patient a change of position.
10. Assist handicapped patients with shaving.
11. Always move or turn patient toward you.

CARE OF EQUIPMENT

1. Remove soiled linen and place in hamper.
2. Wash equipment, rinse, dry and put away.

6. MAKING AN UNOCCUPIED BED

PURPOSE

To provide a clean, comfortable bed.
To provide a neat appearance to the ward.

EQUIPMENT

Two sheets
Plastic mattress cover
Blanket
Plastic pillow cover
Pillowcase
Protective draw sheet or disposable pads, if indicated

PROCEDURE

1. Place mattress cover on mattress. Where necessary and available, plastic mattress covers are used.
2. Place center fold of sheet in center of bed, narrow hem even with foot of bed.
3. Fold excess sheet under the mattress at head of bed.
4. Miter corner.
    a. Pick up hanging sheet 12 inches from head of bed.
    b. Tuck lower corner under mattress.
    c. Bring triangle down over side of bed.
    d. Tuck sheet under mattress.
5. Pull bottom sheet tight and tuck under side of mattress.
6. If draw sheets are indicated, place in center of bed as illustrated. Tuck excess under mattress.
    a. Linen draw sheet is made by folding a regular bed sheet in half - hem to hem.
7. Place center fold of second sheet in center of bed, with hem even with the top of mattress.
8. Tuck excess under foot of mattress.
9. Center fold blanket in middle of bed 6 inches from top of mattress.
10. Fold excess under foot of mattress.
11. Make mitered corner.

MAKING AN UNOCCUPIED BED (Continued)

PROCEDURE (Continued)

12. Place bedspread on bed, center fold in middle of bed even with the top of the mattress. Fold under blanket.
13. Fold cuff of top sheet over bedspread at head of bed.
14. Tuck excess spread under foot of mattress.
15. Miter corner at foot of mattress.
16. Go to other side of bed and follow steps 3 to 15.
17. Place plastic cover on pillow.
18. Place pillow case on pillow.
19. Place pillow on bed with seams at head of bed, open end away from the entrance to the ward.

POINTS TO EMPHASIZE

1. Woolen blankets are to be used only when cotton blankets are not available.
2. Never use woolen blankets when oxygen therapy is in use.
3. Use protective draw sheet or protective pads when indicated.

MITERED CORNER

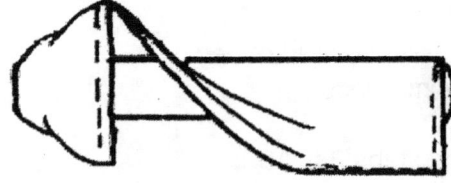

Pick up hanging sheet 12 inches from head of bed.

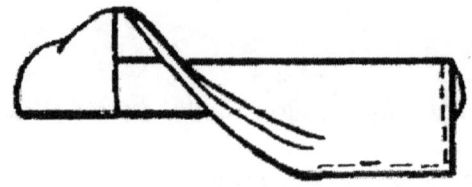

Tuck lower corner under mattress.

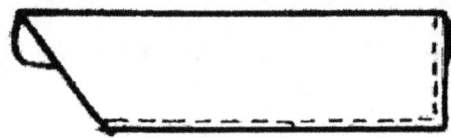

Bring triangle down over side of bed.

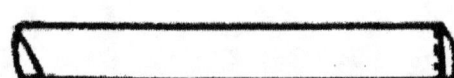

Tuck sheet under mattress.

COMPLETING FOUNDATION
APPLY DRAW SHEETS

1. PLACE RUBBER DRAW SHEET IN CENTER OF BED

2. TUCK EXCESS RUBBER DRAW SHEET IN ON NEAR SIDE OF MATTRESS

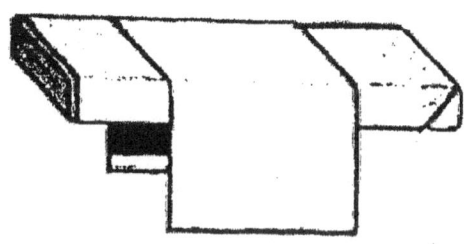

3. PLACE COTTON DRAW SHEET OVER RUBBER DRAW SHEET

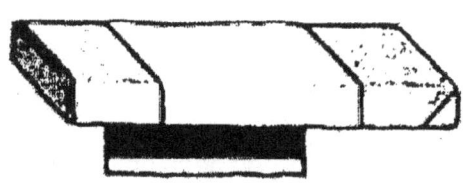

4. TUCK EXCESS COTTON DRAW SHEET IN ON NEAR SIDE OF MATTRESS

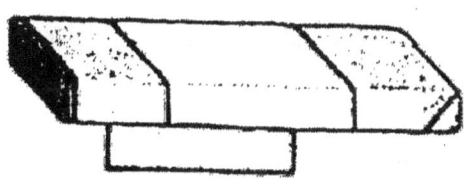

5. TUCK EXCESS RUBBER DRAW SHEET IN ON OPPOSITE SIDE OF MATTRESS

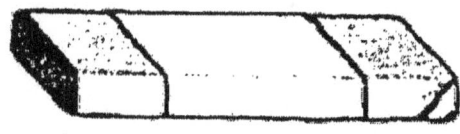

6. TUCK EXCESS COTTON DRAW SHEET IN ON OPPOSITE SIDE OF MATTRESS

7. MAKING AN OCCUPIED BED

PURPOSE

To provide clean linen with least exertion to patient.
To refresh patient.
To prevent pressure sores.

EQUIPMENT

Two sheets
Pillowcase
Blanket
Protective draw sheet or disposable pads, if indicated
Hamper

PROCEDURE

1. Place chair at foot of bed.
2. Push bedside locker away from bed.
3. Pull mattress to head of bed.
4. Loosen all bedding.
5. Remove pillow and place on chair.
6. Remove bedspread by folding from top to bottom, pick up in center and place on back of chair.
7. Remove blanket in same manner.
8. Turn patient to one side of the bed.
9. If cotton draw sheet is used, roll draw sheet close to patient's back.
10. Turn back protective sheet over patient.
11. Roll bottom sheet close to patient's back.
12. Straighten mattress cover as necessary.
13. Place clean sheet on bed with the center fold in the middle and narrow hem even with foot of bed.
14. Tuck in excess at head of bed. Miter corner and tuck in at side.
15. Bring down protective sheet; straighten and tuck in.
16. Make draw sheet by folding a sheet from hem to hem with smooth side out.
17. Place on bed with fold toward head of bed. Tuck in.

MAKING AN OCCUPIED BED (Continued)

PROCEDURE (Continued)

18. Roll patient over to completed side of bed.
19. Go to other side of the bed.
20. Remove soiled sheets and place in hamper.
21. Check soiled linen for personal articles.
22. Turn back draw sheets over patient.
23. Pull bottom sheet tight and smooth.
24. Pull protective sheet and draw sheet tight and smooth.
25. Bring patient to center of bed.
26. Place top sheet over patient, wide hem even with top of mattress.
27. Ask patient to hold clean top sheet.
28. Remove soiled top sheet. Place in hamper.
29. Place blanket 6 inches from top of mattress.
30. Make pleat in sheet and blanket over patient's toes.
31. Tuck in excess at foot of bed and miter corners.
32. Place bedspread on bed even with top of mattress. Fold under blanket.
33. Fold sheet over bedspread and blanket at head of bed.
34. Tuck in excess bedspread at foot of bed. Miter corners. Allow triangle to hang loosely.
35. Put clean pillowcase on pillow. Place under patient's head with closed end toward entrance to ward.
36. Adjust bed as desired by patient.
37. Straighten unit. Leave bedside stand within reach of patient.

POINTS TO EMPHASIZE

1. Always turn patient toward you to prevent possibility of injury and/or falls.
2. Make sure that foundation sheets are smooth and dry.

MAKING AN OCCUPIED BED

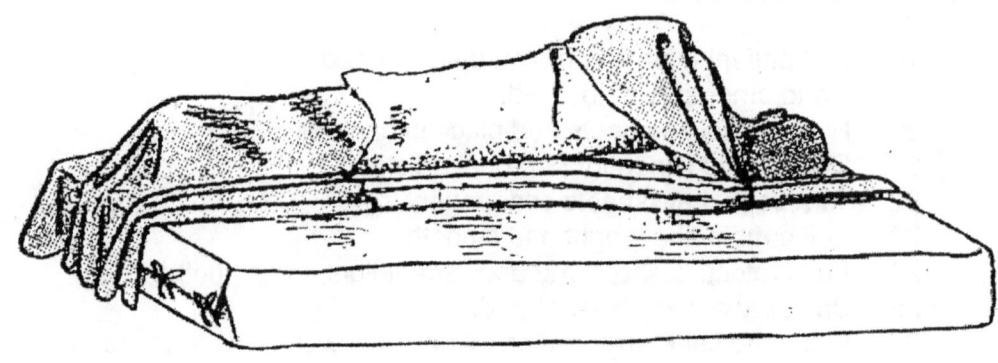

**TURN PATIENT TOWARD YOU
FAN FOLD SOILED LINEN
AGAINST PATIENTS BACK**

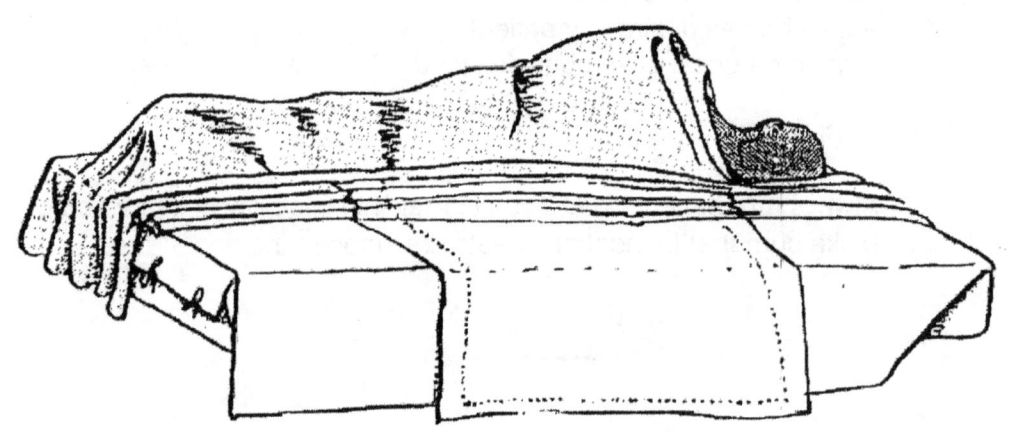

**MAKE UP ONE HALF THE BED
BOTTOM SHEET, THEN
RUBBER DRAW SHEET**

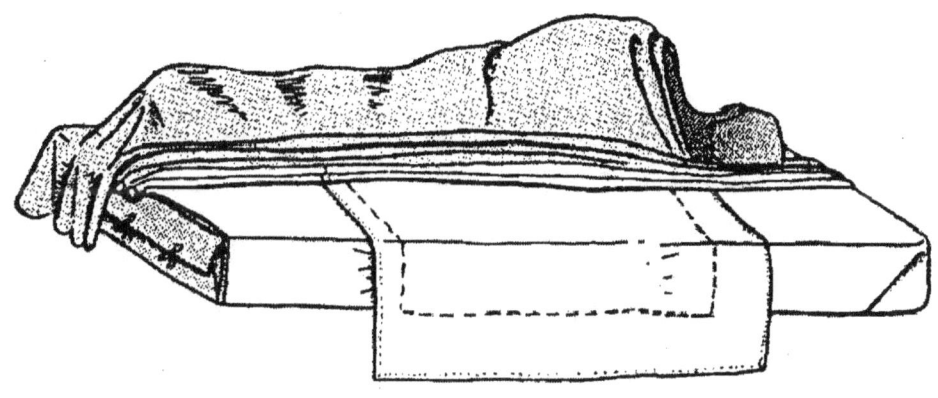

ADD COTTON DRAW SHEET

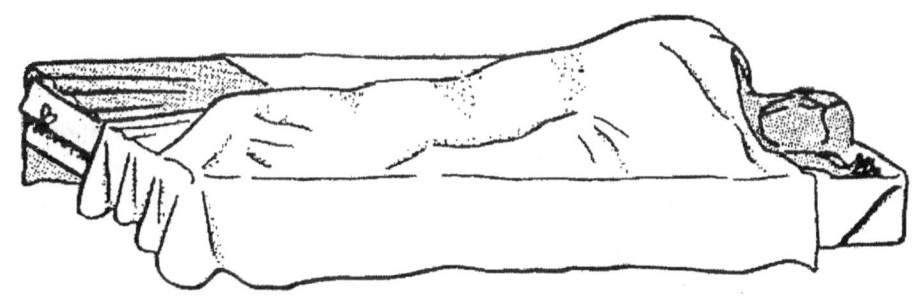

TURN PATIENT ONTO CLEAN LINEN
MAKE OPPOSITE SIDE OF BED

8. SERVING DIETS FROM FOOD CART

PURPOSE

To provide an attractively served food tray for a patient in a hospital where central food tray service is not available.

EQUIPMENT

Cart with food
Cart with trays, dishes, silver, and serving utensils

PROCEDURE

1. Clear the patient's bedside or overbed table.
2. Place table within patient's reach.
3. Place patient in a comfortable position.
4. Wash hands. Wheel food and tray carts to the unit.
5. Place beverage, salad, soup and dessert on the tray.
6. Fill glasses, cups and bowls three fourths full.
7. Serve small portions of hot food in an attractive manner.
8. Check diet list for type of diet each patient is to receive.
9. Carry tray and place it in a convenient position for the patient. Help the patient with the food if necessary.
10. After patient has finished, note how much he has eaten. Collect tray and return to main galley.

POINTS TO EMPHASIZE

1. The ward should be quiet and in readiness for meals.
2. Serve hot food hot and cold food cold.
3. Ice cream, sherbert and jello are kept in the refrigerator until ready to serve.
4. Do not hurry patient.
5. Do not smoke while working with food.
6. Refer to Special Diet Manual for special diet information.
7. Check visible file to determine if patient may have regular diet.
8. Make rounds to check that every patient has been served and received the correct diet.

SERVING DIETS FROM FOOD CART (Continued)

CARE OF EQUIPMENT WHERE MAIN GALLEY DOES NOT HAVE DISH WASHING FACILITIES

1. Scrape and stack dishes:
    a. Solid food into garbage can.
    b. Liquids into drain.
2. Clean and stack trays.
3. Wash dishes with hot soapy water. Stack in dish sterilizer.
4. Follow instructions on sterilizer. Temperature of final rinse water 180° F. Allow to air dry. Put away.
5. Place trays on cart with tray cover, silver and napkins. Salt, pepper, sugar go on all trays except Special Diets.
6. Clean food cart. Return to main galley.

9. CENTRAL TRAY SERVICE

PURPOSE

To provide attractively served food to the patient in an efficient manner.

PROCEDURE

1. Check list of patients who are not permitted food or fluids by mouth.
2. Clear bedside or overbed table.
3. Place table within reach of patient.
4. Place patient in comfortable position.
5. Wash hands. Wheel cart with trays to unit.
6. Take tray from cart and check to see if it is complete.
7. Read tray card.
8. See that tray is served to patient listed on the selective menus or the Special Diet Request that is placed on each tray.
9. Call each patient by name or check his identification band. Place his tray within easy reach.
10. Feed patient or assist him as necessary such as buttering his bread, cutting his meat, etc. Allow patient to do as much for himself as possible.
11. Make rounds to check that each patient entitled to a tray has been fed. The Diet List may be used as a check off list.
12. After the patient has finished eating, collect tray immediately and return to cart. Make a note of food eaten and record on Intake and Output Sheet as indicated.
13. Report all complaints about food to Food Service.

POINTS TO EMPHASIZE

1. Serve trays promptly.
2. Do not hurry patient.
3. Make rounds to check that all patients have been fed.

10. CARE OF ICE MACHINE AND HANDLING OF ICE, BEDSIDE PITCHERS, AND GLASSES

PURPOSE

To prevent ice machines from becoming a source of infection due to cross-contamination.

EQUIPMENT

To clean and disinfect ice machine:
- Clean gloves, disposable
- 4x4 sponges
- Scouring powder
- Sodium hypochlorite
- Clean 1 gallon container
- Clean ice scoop

PROCEDURE

1. Disconnect ice machine from electrical outlet.
2. Wash hands.
3. Use ice scoop to dispose of any existing ice. Pour tap water into ice storage compartment to melt any remaining ice.
4. Put on gloves and remove scale and other debris with 4x4 sponges and scouring powder.
5. Rinse thoroughly with tap water.
6. Place 1/2 ounce of sodium hypocholrite in 1 gallon of water.
7. Using 4 x 4's wipe all accessible areas of interior with sodium hypochlorite solution. Pay particualr attention to ice chute.
8. Repeat step #7.
9. Allow solution to remain in machine for 30 minutes.
10. Rinse thoroughly with clean tap water three times.
11. Clean the exterior of the ice machine.
12. Connect ice machine to electrical outlet.

POINTS TO EMPHASIZE

1. Keep exterior of machine clean between weekly disinfecting of interior.
2. Limit access to ice machine to nursing service personnel.
3. Always keep door closed when not removing ice.
4. Locate ice machine in a "clean" area of the ward or hospital.
5. If ice must be transported, containers should be clean and covered.
6. Use a scoop or tongs when handling ice. Never handle ice with bare hands.
7. Never store the scoop in the ice when not in use.

CARE OF ICE MACHINE AND HANDLING OF ICE, BEDSIDE PITCHERS, AND GLASSES (Continued)

POINTS TO EMPHASIZE (Continued)

8. The scoop or tongs must be sanitized at least daily.
9. Each patient should have his own bedside water pitcher with cover.
10. Glasses used for drinking water should be sent to the kitchen for exchange of clean glasses on a routine basis.
11. Culture ice machines according to local hospital policy and record in ice culture log.

CARE OF EQUIPMENT

1. Discard disposable equipment.
2. Replace cleaning gear.

11. FEEDING THE HELPLESS PATIENT

PURPOSE

To promote adequate nutrition of the helpless patient.
To encourage self-help when condition permits.

PROCEDURE

1. Place the patient in a sitting position unless otherwise ordered.
2. Place a towel across the patient's chest. Tuck a napkin under his chin.
3. Place tray on overbed table or bedside stand.
4. Give the patient a piece of buttered bread if he is able to hold it.
5. Feed the patient in the order in which he likes to be fed.
6. Offer liquids during the meal. Have patient use a drinking tube if necessary.
7. Give a small amount of food at one time. Allow the patient to chew and swallow food before offering him more. Do not rush your patient.
8. If patient is inclined to talk, talk with him.
9. Note amount of food he has taken. Record amount of fluid if on measured intake and output.
10. Remove tray. Leave patient comfortable.

POINTS TO EMPHASIZE

1. As you are feeding a blind patient tell him what you are offering and whether it is hot or cold.
2. Encourage a blind patient to begin feeding himself as soon as he is able and when indicated.
3. When encouraging a blind patient to feed himself, arrange tray the same way each time. Place foods on plate in the same clockwise direction and fill glasses and cups one-half full to avoid spilling.
4. If patient has difficulty in swallowing, have oral suction machine at bedside.

12. EVENING CARE

PURPOSE

To relax and prepare patient for the night.
To observe the patient's condition.

EQUIPMENT

Basin of warm water
Towel, washcloth and soap
Toothbrush, and dentifrice/mouthwash
Curved basin
Glass of water
Rubbing alcohol/skin lotion
Comb

PROCEDURE

1. Offer bedpan and urinal.
2. Give oral hygiene.
3. Wash patient's face and hands.
4. Wash back. Give back rub. Comb hair.
5. Straighten and tighten bottom sheets.
6. Freshen pillows.
7. Place extra blanket at foot of bed if weather is cool.
8. Make provision for ventilation of unit.
9. Clean and straighten unit and remove excess gear.

POINTS TO EMPHASIZE

1. Indicated for all bed patients and those on limited activity.
2. Change soiled linen as necessary.
3. Patient may assist with care as condition permits.
4. Ask the patient if soap may be used on the face.
5. Screen patients who require the use of bedpan.

13. CARE OF THE SERIOUSLY ILL PATIENT

PURPOSE

To provide optimum care and close observation of the seriously ill patient.
To keep the patient mentally and physically comfortable.

EQUIPMENT

Special mouth care tray
Rubbing alcohol/skin lotion
Bed linen as necessary
Pillow and/or supporting appliances
Special equipment as needed:

- I.V. Standard
- Suction machine
- Oxygen
- Drainage bottles
- Intake and Output work sheet

PROCEDURE

1. Place patient where he can be easily and <u>closely</u> observed.
2. Keep room quiet, clean and clear of excess gear.
3. Bathe patient daily and P.R.N.
4. Maintain good oral hygiene every 2-4 hours.
5. Wash, rub back and change position every 2 hours unless contraindicated.
6. Speak to patient in a calm, natural tone of voice even if he appears to be unconscious.
7. Report any sudden change in condition.
8. Keep an accurate intake and output record if ordered.
9. Offer fluids if patient is conscious and is able to take them.
10. Record and Report:
    a. Changes in T.P.R. and blood pressure.
    b. State of consciousness.
    c. All observations.

CARE OF THE SERIOUSLY ILL PATIENT (Continued)

POINTS TO EMPHASIZE

1. All patients are seen by a chaplain when they are placed on the Serious or Very Seriously ill list.
2. Be considerate and kind to the patient's relatives.
3. Keep charting up-to-date.
4. Do not discuss patient's condition when the conversation might be overheard by the patient or unauthorized persons.
5. Refer all questions concerning the patient's condition to the doctor or nurse.
6. Be sure all procedures for placing a patient on the SL or VSL have been completed; for exmaple, inventory of personal effects and valuables.

COMMON DIAGNOSTIC NORMS

CONTENTS

		Page
1.	Respiration	1
2.	Pulse-Rate	1
3.	Blood Pressure	1
4.	Blood Metabolism	1
5.	Blood	1
6.	Urine	3
7.	Spinal Fluid	4
8.	Snellen Chart Fractions	4

COMMON DIAGNOSTIC NORMS

1. RESPIRATION: From 16-20 per minute.

2. PULSE-RATE: Men, about 72 per minute.
   Women, about 80 per minute.

3. BLOOD PRESSURE:
   Men: 110-135 (Systolic)   Women: 95-125   (Systolic)
         70-85   (Diastolic)   65-70   (Diastolic)

4. BASAL METABOLISM: Represents the body energy expended to maintain respiration, circulation, etc. Normal rate ranges from plus 10 to minus 10.

5. BLOOD:

   a. Red Blood (Erythrocyte) Count:
   Male adult - 5,000,000 per cu. mm.
   Female adult - 4,500,000 per cu. mm.
   (Increased in polycythemia vera, poisoning by carbon monoxide, in chronic pulmonary artery sclerosis, and in concentration of blood by sweating, vomiting, or diarrhea.)
   (Decreased in pernicious anemia, secondary anemia, and hypochronic anemia.)
   b. White Blood (Leukocyte) Count: 6,000 to 8,000 per cu. mm.
   (Increased with muscular exercise, acute infections, intestinal obstruction, coronary thrombosis, leukemias.)
   (Decreased due to injury to source of blood formation and interference in delivery of cells to bloodstream, typhoid, pernicious anemia, arsenic and benzol poisoning.)
   The total leukocyte group is made up of a number of diverse varieties of white blood cells. Not only the total leukocyte count, but also the relative count of the diverse varieties, is an important aid to diagnosis. In normal blood, from:
   70-72% of the leukocytes are *polymorphonuclear neuirophils.*
   2-4% of the leukocytes are *polymorphonuclear eosinophils.*
   0-.5% of the leukocytes are *basophils,*
   20-25% of the leukocytes are *lymphocytes.*
   2-6% of the leukocytes are *monocytes.*
   c. Blood Platelet (Thrombocyte) Count:
   250,000 per cu. mm. Blood platelets are important in blood coagulation.

   d. Hemoglobin Content:
   May normally vary from 85-100%. A 100% hemoglobin content is equivalent to the presence of 15.6 grams of hemoglobin in 100 c.c. of blood.
   e. Color Index:
   Represents the relative amount of hemoglobin contained in a red blood corpuscle compared with that of a normal individual of the patient's age and sex.
   The normal is 1. To determine the color index, the percentage of hemoglobin is divided by the ratio of red cells in the patient's blood to a norm of 5,000,000. Thus, a hemoglobin content of 60% and a red cell count of 4,000,000 (80% of 5,000,000) produces an abnormal color index of .75.

f. Sedimentation Rate:
Represents the measurement of the speed with which red cells settle toward the bottom of a containing vessel. The rate is expressed in millimeters per hour, and indicates the total sedimentation of red blood cells at the end of 60 minutes.

Average rate:	4-7 mm. in 1 hour
Slightly abnormal rate:	8-15 mm. in 1 hour
Moderately abnormal rate:	16-40 mm. in 1 hour
Considerably abnormal rate:	41-80 mm. in 1 hour

(The sedimentation rate is above normal in patients with chronic infections, or in whom there is a disease process involving destruction of tissue, such as coronary thrombosis, etc.)

g. Blood Sugar:
90-120 mg. per 100 c.c. (Normal)
In mild diabetics: 150-300 mg. per 100 c.c.
In severe diabetics: 300-1200 mg. per 100 c.c.

h. Blood Lead:
0.1 mg. or less in 100 c.c. (Normal). Greatly increased in lead poisoning.

i. Non-Protein Nitrogen:
Since the function of the kidneys is to remove from the blood certain of the waste products of cellular activity, any degree of accumulation of these waste products in the blood is a measure of renal malfunction. For testing purposes, the substances chosen for measurement are the nitrogen-containing products of protein combustion, their amounts being estimated in terms of the nitrogen they contain. These substances are urea, uric acid, and creatinine, the sum total of which, in addition to any traces of other waste products, being designated as total non-protein nitrogen (NPN).

The normal limits of NPN in 100 c.c. of blood range from 25-40 mg. Of this total, urea nitrogen normally constitutes 12-15 mg., uric acid 2-4 mg., and creatinine 1-2 mg.

6. URINE:

   a. Urine - Lead:
   0.08 mg. per liter of urine (normal).
   (Increased in lead poisoning.)

   b. Sugar:
   From none to a faint trace (normal).
   From 0.5% upwards (abnormal).
   (Increased in diabetes mellitus.)

   c. Urea:
   Normal excretion ranges from 15-40 grams in 24 hours.
   (Increased in fever and toxic states.)

   d. Uric Acid:
   Normal excretion is variable. (Increased in leukemia and gout.)

   e. Albumin:
   Normal renal cells allow a trace of albumin to pass into the urine, but this trace is so minute that it cannot be detected by ordinary tests.

f. Casts:
In some abnormal conditions, the kidney tubules become lined with substances which harden and form a mould or *oast* inside the tubes. These are later washed out by the urine, and may be detected microscopically. They are named either from the substance composing them, or from their appearance. Thus, there are pus casts, epithelial casts from the walls of the tubes, hyaline casts formed from coagulable elements of the blood, etc.

g. Pus Cells:
These are found in the urine in cases of nephritis or other inflammatory conditions of the urinary tract.

h. Epithelial Cells:
These are always present in the urine. Their number is greatly multiplied, however, in inflammatory conditions of the urinary tract.

i. Specific Gravity:
This is the ratio between the weight of a given volume of urine to that of the same volume of water. A normal reading ranges from 1.015 to 1.025. A high specific gravity usually occurs in diabetes mellitus. A low specific gravity is associated with a polyuria.

7. SPINAL FLUID:

   a. Spinal Fluid Pressure (Manometric Reading):
   100-200 mm. of water or 7-15 mm, of mercury (normal).
   (Increased in cerebral edema, cerebral hemorrhage, meningitis, certain brain tumors, or if there is some process blocking the fluid circulation in the spinal column, such as a tumor or herniated nucleus pulposus impinging on the spinal canal.)

   b. Quickenstedt's Sign:
   When the veins in the neck are compressed on one or both sides, there is a rapid rise in the pressure of the cerebrospinal fluid of healthy persons, and this rise quickly disappears when pressure is removed from the neck. But when there is a block of the vertebral canal, the pressure of the cerebrospinal fluid is little or not at all affected by this maneuver.

   c. Cerebrospinal Sugar:
   50-60 mg. per 100 c.c. of spinal fluid (normal).
   (Increased in epidemic encephalitis, diabetes mellitus, and increased intracranial pressure.)
   (Decreased in purulent and tuberculous meningitis.)

   d. Cerebrospinal Protein:
   15-40 mg. per 100 c.c. of spinal fluid (normal).
   (Increased in suppurative meningitis, epileptic seizures, cerebrospinal syphilis, anterior poliomyelitis, brain abscess, and brain tumor.)

   e. Colloidal Gold Test:
   This test is made to determine the presence of cerebrospinal protein.

   f. Cerebrospinal Cell Count:
   0-10 lymphocytes per cu. mm. (normal).

   g. Cerebrospinal Globulin:
   Normally negative. It is positive in various types of meningitis, various types of syphilis of the central nervous system, in poliomyelitis, in brain tumor, and in intracranial hemorrhage.

8. **SNELLEN CHART FRACTIONS AS SCHEDULE LOSS DETERMINANTS:**

   a. Visual acuity is expressed by a Snell Fraction, where the numerator represents the distance, in feet, between the subject and the test chart, and the denominator represents the distance, in feet, at which a normal eye could read a type size which the abnormal eye can read only at 20 feet.
   b. Thus, 20/20 means that an individual placed 20 feet from the test chart clearly sees the size of type that one with normal vision should see at that distance.
   c. 20/60 means that an individual placed 20 feet from the test chart can read only a type size, at a distance of 20 feet, which one of normal vision could read at 60 feet.
   d. Reduction of a Snellen Fraction to its simplest form roughly indicates the amount of vision remaining in an eye. Thus, a visual acuity of 20/60 corrected implies a useful vision of 1/3 or 33 1/3%, and a visual loss of 2/3 or 66 2/3% of the eye.

   Similarly:

Visual Acuity (Corrected)	Percentage Loss of Use of Eye
20/20	No loss
20/25	20%
20/30	33 1/3%
20/40	50%
20/50	60%
20/60	66 2/3%
20/70	70% (app.)
20/80	75%
20/100	100% (since loss of 80% or more constitutes industrial blindness)

www.ingramcontent.com/pod-product-compliance
Lightning Source LLC
Chambersburg PA
CBHW081813300426
44116CB00014B/2346